INSTITUTE OF PSYCHIATRY

Maudsley Monographs

MAUDSLEY MONOGRAPHS

HENRY MAUDSLEY, from whom the series of monographs takes its name, was the founder of the Maudsley Hospital and the most prominent English psychiatrist of his generation. Maudsley Hospital was united with the Bethlem Royal Hospital in 1948, and its medical school, renamed the Institute of Psychiatry at the same time, became a constituent part of the British Postgraduate Medical Federation. It is entrusted by the University of London with the duty to advance psychiatry by teaching and research.

The monograph series reports work carried out in the Institute and in the associated Hospital. Some of the monographs are directly concerned with clinical problems; others, less obviously relevant, are in scientific fields that are cultivated for the furtherance of psychiatry.

Joint Editors

Professor Gerald Russell
MD, FRCP, FRCP (Ed.),
FRC Psych.

Professor Edward Marley
MA, MD, DSc., FRCP,
FRC Psych.

Assistant editor

Dr Paul Williams
MD, MRC Psych., DPM

with assistance of

Miss S. E. Hague, BSc. (Econ), MA

INSTITUTE OF PSYCHIATRY

Maudsley Monographs

Number Thirty-One

The Neuropathology of Temporal Lobe Epilepsy

By

C. J. BRUTON, MD (London), LRCP, MRCS

Neuropathologist; Dept. of Neuropathology, Runwell Hospital, Essex
Division of Psychiatry; CRC Northwick Park Hospital, Harrow, Middlesex
Late Senior Registrar, Dept. of Neuropathology, Runwell Hospital, Essex
and Dept. of Neuropathology, Institute of Psychiatry

OXFORD UNIVERSITY PRESS

1988

Oxford University Press, Walton Street, Oxford OX2 6DP

Oxford New York Toronto
Delhi Bombay Calcutta Madras Karachi
Petaling Jaya Singapore Hong Kong Tokyo
Nairobi Dar es Salaam Cape Town
Melbourne Auckland

and associated companies in
Berlin Ibadan

Oxford is a trade mark of Oxford University Press

Published in the United States
by Oxford University Press, New York

British Library Cataloguing in Publication Data
Bruton, C. J.
The neuropathology of temporal lobe
epilepsy.—(Maudsley monographs ; no. 31)
1. Temporal lobe epilepsy
I. Title. II. University of London.
Institute of Psychiatry III. Series
616.8'5307   RC 372.5
ISBN 0 19 712155 1

Library of Congress Cataloging in Publication Data
Bruton, C. J.
The neuropathology of temporal lobe epilepsy / C. J. Bruton.
p.   cm.—(Maudsley monographs ; no. 31)
Bibliography: p.   Includes index.
1. Temporal lobe epilepsy—Pathophysiology.   2. Temporal lobe
epilepsy—Surgery.   I. Title.   II. Series.
[DNLM: 1. Epilepsy, Temporal Lobe—pathology.   2. Temporal Lobe—
surgery.   W1 MA997 no. 31 / WL 385 B913n]
RC372.5.B78   1988   616.8'53—dc19   87–31339
ISBN 0 19 712155 1

Set by Latimer Trend & Company Ltd, Plymouth
Printed in Great Britain by
Butler & Tanner Ltd, Frome, Somerset

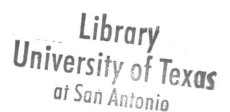

Preface

From earliest times the physicians who studied epilepsy sought to discover the origins of the disorder. Indeed, one volume of the Hippocratic Collection of Medical Writings (400 BC) is devoted to *The Sacred Disease*. However, although the major convulsive forms of epilepsy were relatively easy to document, it was only a century ago that Hughlings Jackson, using the anatomical theory of Broca and the experimental work of Ferrier, described an association between a peculiar 'dreamy state' form of epilepsy and visible abnormalities in the temporal lobe of the brain.

At the same time, Victor Horsley had performed the first neurosurgical operation designed specifically to relieve epileptic fits. While Horsley operated, Hughlings Jackson and Ferrier looked on (Taylor, 1987), a triumvirate of neuroscientists whose efforts placed both epilepsy surgery and 'dreamy state' or 'temporal lobe' epilepsy firmly on the medical map.

Nevertheless, another 60 years were to pass before a specific surgical operation for temporal lobe epilepsy became feasible following introduction of the first EEG machines which enabled accurate localization of the abnormal electrical impulses in the brain tracings of epileptic patients.

The operation of anterior temporal lobectomy was developed first by Penfield but soon modified by Falconer, who designed an *en bloc* resection which produced a single anatomically intact specimen for examination by the neuropathologist. For the next 25 years, Falconer and his colleagues at the Neurosurgical Unit of Guy's, Maudsley, and King's College Hospitals were at the forefront of temporal lobe surgery as a treatment for patients with severe temporal lobe fits.

This monograph is a shortened version of an MD thesis presented to London University in 1984. It is a clinico-pathological survey of 249 cases of anterior temporal lobectomy performed by Mr. Murray Falconer in the 25 years beginning January 1st 1950. The aims of the study were to classify the various abnormalities found in the brain tissue removed from the epileptic patients and to identify, if possible, those patients most likely to benefit from surgery.

The results have been encouraging in that it has proved possible not only to develop a revised system of classification which highlights certain differences between the various types of abnormality but also to construct a 'league table' of benefit from the operation which may be of use to clinicians who deal with these cases.

REFERENCE

Taylor, D. C. (1987). *Surgical treatment of the epilepsies* (ed. Engel J. Jr.), pp. 7–11. Raven Press, New York.

Wickford   C.J.B.
January 1988

Acknowledgements

The material for this study was collected diligently over many years by a large number of people. It represents almost a lifetime's effort and enthusiasm by a highly skilled neurosurgeon, the late Mr. Murray Falconer; I hope the results go some way to vindicate his attempts to help some of the most severely afflicted temporal lobe epileptics.

The work also represents part of the massive contribution to neuropathology made by Professor J. A. N. Corsellis, with whom I have been privileged to work for nearly 20 years. I am greatly indebted to Professor Corsellis, not only for the overall direction of this project, but also for his friendship and support throughout the years.

I am also greatly indebted to Professor Peter Lantos for his kindness in giving time so freely to read and discuss the manuscript in all stages of its production.

Substantial statistical advice was received from Mr. Keith Miller, late of Runwell Hospital and of the Institute of Psychiatry, and Mr. Nigel Colter of the Division of Psychiatry, C.R.C., Northwick Park Hospital. I thank Keith for his support and for his interpretation of the otherwise incomprehensible data which emerged from the Institute's computer, and Nigel for explaining and charting the final statistical results.

I would like to thank Professor David Taylor for his help and advice with the clinical material and for giving me the opportunity to visit him in Manchester on the very day when that city received its largest single day's rainfall since records began.

Mrs. Edwina Perkins and Mrs. Barbara Bullman have typed the manuscript with great efficiency and speed, while coping magnificently with the introduction of modern computer technology. I thank them for all their efforts.

On the technical side, Rosemary Brown, Miss E. Whitehall and Valerie Gray have prepared the histology slides with expertise. They have shown me great friendship and kindness, personally and professionally, over the years, and I am very grateful to all three.

I am also indebted to Dr. Luis Carrasco and Valerie Gray, who produced the various macro and micro photographs and answered my questions with patience and understanding.

Finally, I send thanks to the many unnamed colleagues at Runwell Hospital and at the Institute of Psychiatry who have helped to make this survey possible. Any errors are mine.

Contents

Tables

Figures

1. Introduction

Although most types of epileptic seizure were described clearly in the earliest medical literature, it was only a hundred years ago that Hughlings Jackson, in two classic clinico-pathological papers, revealed the true nature of temporal lobe epilepsy and its common association with localized brain damage (Jackson & Beevor, 1889; Jackson & Coleman, 1898).

In the present century a revived interest in temporal lobe function (Papez, 1937), combined with the introduction of electroencephalography, led to the identification of abnormal electrical discharges in epileptic subjects, and in particular to one type of paroxysmal abnormality which was thought to be characteristic of 'psychomotor' or temporal lobe attacks (Gibbs, Gibbs & Lennox, 1937; Jasper and Kershman, 1941). Thus for the first time electrical abnormality over the temporal lobes could be identified with some accuracy and this, combined with the development of neurosurgery and difficulties in the medical treatment of certain patients with temporal lobe epilepsy, led to the surgical removal of such lobes in order to help the most severely affected patients (Penfield & Flanigin, 1950; Jasper, Pertuisset and Flanigin, 1951; Bailey & Gibbs, 1951).

The earliest operations followed the method designed by Penfield in Montreal in which variable amounts of the temporal lobe were sucked out in fragments – a method, however, which made subsequent anatomical and neuropathological assessment of the lobe difficult (Earle, Baldwin & Penfield, 1953; Meyer, Falconer & Beck, 1954; Jensen, 1975(a); Bruton, 1984).

In Britain, however, Falconer developed the method of *en bloc* resection which helped greatly with the subsequent anatomical orientation of the lobe and its histological examination. A steady flow of observations followed on the clinical, electroencephalographic, psychiatric, and neuropathological aspects of temporal lobe surgery (Meyer, Falconer & Beck, 1954; Falconer, Hill, Meyer, Mitchell & Pond, 1955; Falconer, Driver & Serafetinides, 1962; Falconer, Serafetinides & Corsellis, 1964; Taylor & Falconer, 1968).

From a neuropathological point of view it soon became clear that about two-thirds of the resected temporal lobes contained an identifiable abnormality, which was most commonly a hardened or sclerotic hippocampus (Meyer, Falconer & Beck, 1954). The lesion, known variously as incisural sclerosis, hippocampal sclerosis, Ammon's horn sclerosis or mesial temporal sclerosis (Earle, Baldwin & Penfield, 1953; Meyer, Falconer & Beck, 1954; Margerison & Corsellis, 1966) was similar to that recorded earlier in many classic post-mortem studies of non-operated patients with chronic idiopathic epilepsy. This gave rise to a discussion concerning, first, its relationship to the clinical and the EEG findings in temporal lobectomy patients (Crome, 1955; Margerison & Corsellis, 1966) and, secondly, its association with febrile convulsions (Cavanagh & Meyer, 1956; Falconer, Serafetinides & Corsellis, 1964; Falconer, 1968) and with birth injury (Earle, Baldwin & Penfield, 1953; Ounsted, Lindsay & Norman, 1966; Veith, 1970).

More recently, well-controlled animal experiments involving induced seizures have not only replicated Ammon's horn pathology but have also begun to identify some of the complex physiological factors needed to produce the damage (Meldrum & Brierley, 1973; Meldrum, Vigouroux & Brierley, 1973; Meldrum, 1983). From these results the authors have postulated that damage to the hippocampus in epilepsy may be due to metabolic changes in overactive neurons, and in particular to the effects of excessive intracellular calcium ion entry into the rapidly firing nerve cells, and that lesions caused by failing energy production do not appear until severe degrees of hypoxia are reached. It would appear that these acute lesions, when present, gradually 'ripen' (Earle, Baldwin & Penfield, 1953) into scar tissue so that sooner or later the effect may be to disrupt normal cerebral activity by giving rise to a tendency to further epileptic attacks.

In contrast to the considerable interest centred on the problem of Ammon's horn sclerosis there has been much less emphasis on those patients whose resected temporal lobes show no such pathology. Most studies have found that about 20 per cent of all lobes contain a small focal lesion, whereas many of the remainder appear histologically normal or have some minor ill-defined abnormality which may be classed as 'equivocal' − or as 'no significant lesion' (Falconer, Hill, Meyer, Mitchell & Pond, 1955; Jann Brown, 1973).

The small focal lesions are composed of a miscellany of 'tumours', developmental anomalies, post-traumatic scars or partly healed abscess cavities, and are known by an equal miscellany of names (Falconer, Pond, Meyer & Woolf, 1953; Cavanagh, 1958; Taylor, Falconer, Bruton & Corsellis, 1971). However, there have been few studies of their relative incidence, nature and distribution and no detailed study of the equivocal lesions or of those patients in whom no visible abnormality has been detected even though some of these cases appear to benefit from surgery (Falconer & Serafetinides, 1963; Falconer, Serafetinides & Corsellis, 1964).

Against this background the time seemed appropriate to reinvestigate all the available material from the cases of temporal lobe epilepsy which were operated upon by Mr. Murray Falconer during the 25 years from January 1950, when he developed the *en bloc* method of anterior temporal lobectomy, paying particular attention not only to the neuropathological abnormalities, but also to their classification and to the long-term effects of surgery.

The results of the investigation were presented in the form of a thesis (Bruton, 1984) and the present monograph is an attempt to crystallize the more pertinent findings, especially those relating to the long-term effect of surgery according to the different types of abnormality in the temporal lobe.

2. Materials and method of study

The 249 patients in this study suffered from intractable temporal lobe epilepsy and were referred as possible candidates for surgery to the Neurosurgical Unit of the Guy's, Maudsley, and King's College Hospitals during the 25 years beginning January 1st, 1950.

CLINICAL INVESTIGATIONS

On arrival at the Unit all patients underwent a full clinical, neurological, and psychiatric assessment. Relatives were interviewed and summaries were made of the notes from other hospitals. Details of the fit pattern, types of aura, duration of epilepsy, and previous treatment were noted, particular attention being paid to the adequacy of medication in the control of fits. Routine blood estimations, skull X-rays, and an air encephalogram were performed and the cerebrospinal fluid was examined. Most patients also underwent bilateral carotid arteriography. In addition, nearly every patient also underwent detailed psychometric investigation which included full scale verbal and performance IQ tests.

ELECTROENCEPHALOGRAPHIC INVESTIGATIONS

Serial electroencephalograms had been made on all patients, often over a period of years. However, in addition to these routine studies, more specialized techniques were sometimes used (Hill, 1953; Pampiglione & Kerridge, 1956). These techniques involved making recordings from needles placed under both temporal lobes (sphenoidal electrodes), and a sleep-recording performed after an intravenous injection of thiopentone.

SELECTION OF PATIENTS FOR OPERATION

Four criteria had to be fulfilled:
1. Epileptic fits had to be frequent (at least one per month) and not controlled by adequate treatment with anticonvulsant drugs.
2. Electroencephalographic studies had to show a unilateral temporal lobe focus of spike discharges. Patients with bilateral temporal lobe foci

were not included unless the spike discharge was clearly predominant over the temporal lobe that was to be later excised.

3. The neuroradiological studies had to show no evidence of a space-occupying lesion. (This criterion was applied on the assumption that a temporal lobe mass, if operable, would be treated best by a total removal of the lesion rather than by anterior temporal lobectomy.)

4. The pre-operative IQ had to be greater than 70. (Patients with an IQ less than 70 were excluded on the presumption that any pathological process found in their brains would be more likely to be diffuse rather than confined to one temporal lobe.)

VARIATIONS IN SELECTION PROCEDURE

A few operations were carried out on patients who did not meet all four criteria. Sometimes, for example, there was particularly strong clinical or radiological evidence of a unilateral temporal lobe abnormality which was considered amenable to surgery. In addition the selection procedure altered gradually during the 25 years of the study as a result of experience obtained from the earlier operations.

Thus at the start patients who had an established psychosis as well as epileptic attacks were accepted for operation. Experience showed, however, that although the neurosurgeon could often relieve the patient's epilepsy he was seldom able to help the psychosis. Therefore cases of this type came to be excluded (Taylor, 1975).

Similar experience showed that the best operative results were obtained in patients in whom the duration of established temporal lobe fits had been relatively short (Falconer, 1965; Jensen, 1975a). With this in mind, younger patients with a shorter clinical history were referred for operation more frequently as the study progressed.

Otherwise the selection procedure remained constant throughout the 25 years.

TEMPORAL LOBE SURGERY

Every patient selected for operation underwent an anterior temporal lobectomy in which the aim was to remove deeper structures such as the hippocampus and amygdaloid nucleus in one block together with the overlying temporal convexity. This technique was developed by Mr. Murray Falconer in order to provide a single anatomically intact specimen for examination by the neuropathologist (Falconer, Hill, Meyer, Mitchell & Pond, 1955). Other surgeons had tended to remove only the area of maximum epileptogenicity (Rasmussen, 1969). These latter techniques provided material which was less satisfactory for neuropathological study (Corsellis, 1970a).

The full operative details have been published by Falconer, Hill, Meyer, Mitchell and Pond (1955) and Falconer (1969).

FOLLOW-UP CARE AND ASSESSMENT

After operation, all patients had a full clinical and neurological examination plus a further IQ test. They were then reviewed by the neurosurgeon within a few weeks and, if possible, at yearly intervals thereafter. When appropriate, they were also referred for psychiatric, psychological or EEG assessment. Some patients have been seen regularly for periods of up to 25 years.

CLINICAL REVIEW

For the purposes of the present investigation all clinical records were made available to the author by kind permission of Mr. C. E. Polkey and Mr. P. Schurr. Using the records, an attempt was made to judge the outcome of the operation by assessing changes in the following features:
1. Fit frequency.
2. Personality and social adjustment.
In each case these changes were graded under four separate headings:
(a) Greatly Improved. (b) Improved. (c) Unaltered. (d) Worse.

DEFINITION OF TERMS

1. Fit frequency

The terminology 'greatly improved' was used only if the patient had been totally fit-free for a period of more than five years after surgery. Thus, by definition, no patient who had been followed up for *less than* five years could be classed as 'greatly improved' even if he had been free of convulsions since operation. The group of 'improved' patients contains all those who had been fit-free for less than five years or in whom the number of fits had been reduced substantially. Assessments were made by reading the daily or weekly fit pattern as mentioned in the patients' records.

2. Personality and social adjustment

In the present review an attempt was made to extract information on the subsequent work record, home life, and marriage, as well as on the mental state and to compare this with the pre-operative data. In addition special attention was paid to three overtly psychiatric features: depression, aggression, and schizophrenia, as these were felt to act as useful indices of normal social integration.

However, the assessment of a 'normal independent life' is much more subjective than the enumeration of the daily number of fits. Nevertheless, importance was placed on such items as a return to full time work, subsequent marriage, living away from institutional care, and so forth, as a general index of normality. Patients were classed as Greatly Improved, Improved, Unaltered or Worse, using the same categories as were chosen for the measurements on fit frequency. There is no denying that the assessments were in some cases more difficult to make than those on fit frequency but after reading the detailed follow-up material accumulated over a period of 10–15 years it was often surprisingly easy to arrive at a justifiable conclusion.

NEUROPATHOLOGY

Naked-eye examination

After operation the resected temporal lobe was fixed in 10% formal-saline for two to three weeks. It was then examined and any relevant abnormalities were photographed. The early specimens were described by members of the staff of the Department of Neuropathology, at the Institute of Psychiatry, under the direction of Professor Alfred Meyer and later of Professor Peter Daniel. After 1960 all lobes have been examined by Doctor J. A. N. Corsellis, either at Runwell Hospital or at the Institute of Psychiatry.

The methods used to describe and record the observations changed during the years of the study. At first some specimens were described only briefly and the extent and localization of any macroscopic lesion was not always pin-pointed precisely. Later, however, they were examined systematically; the lobe was weighed and all macroscopic abnormalities were measured carefully and recorded. The convexity of the lobe was assessed with a note on leptomeninges and cerebral vessels. The deep surface of the lobe was examined, the presence and the extent of the anterior hippocampus in the floor of the temporal horn being a guide to the limits of the surgical resection (Figs. 1, 2, 3a & 3b).

The specimen was then cut into coronal slices, each about 1.0 cm thick (Fig. 4): particular attention was paid to the presence or absence of the hippocampus and amygdaloid nucleus along the medial edge of the lobe.

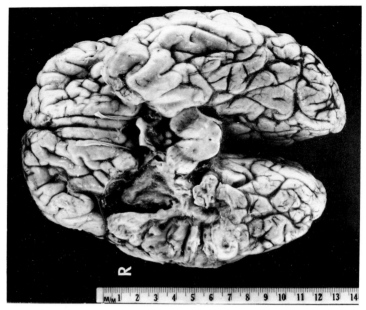

Fig. 1. Case 32. Base of brain with brainstem and cerebellum removed at midbrain level. The right anterior temporal lobe has been resected.

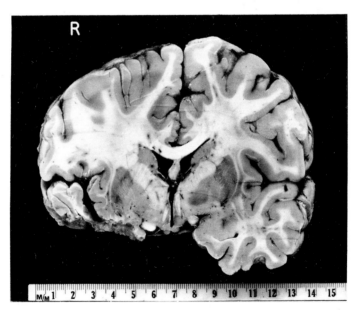

Fig. 2. Case 32. Coronal slice of brain at interventricular foramen level. The right temporal lobe has been removed.

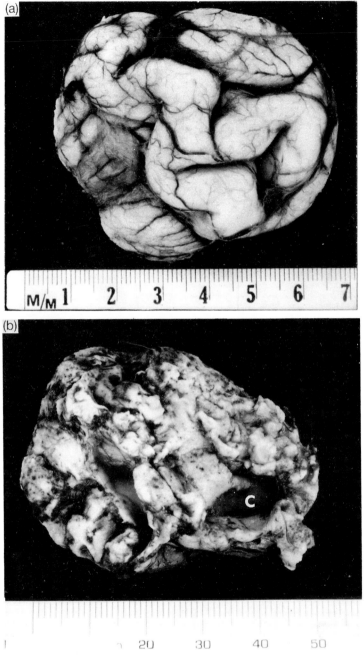

Fig. 3. a. Case 99. Lateral view of resected temporal lobe. b. Case 42. Medial view of resected lobe. Note the cystic cavity 'c' anterior to, but not connected with, the inferior horn of the lateral ventricle.

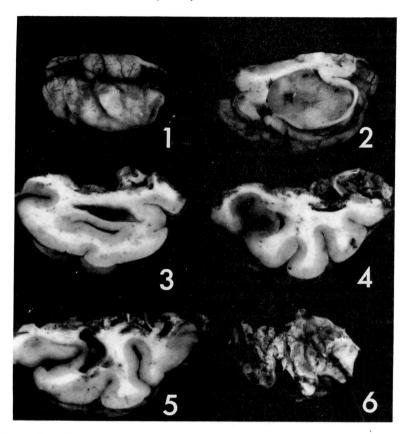

Fig. 4. Case 98. Anterior temporal lobe cut into six coronal slices. Note the Double pathology. Block 2 shows a greyish ovoid mass of abnormal tissue encircled on its edge by a thin rim of cortex. Behind this, in Block 3 there is a cystic cavity in the white matter. A haemorrhagic fragment of hippocampus is visible in Block 4.

TISSUE PROCESSING

Alternate blocks of tissue were taken for embedding in paraffin and in nitrocellulose; blocks for frozen sections were prepared when necessary. Serial sections were cut from selected blocks when necessary. The staining methods used as a routine were Nissl's, using cresyl violet, Heidenhain Woelcke's, for myelin, Mallory's phosphotungstic acid haematoxylin, and van Gieson's stain with iron haematoxylin. The haematoxylin and eosin method and the Gros Bielschowsky techniques for neurofibrils were used routinely on the paraffin-embedded material.

In addition more specialized stains for neuroglia, neutral fats, and so on, were employed when appropriate.

HISTOLOGICAL ASSESSMENT

The histological diagnosis forms the linchpin of the study, and against it all clinical information has been compared. The criteria for histological classification were, therefore, chosen carefully. The diagnostic groups do not conform strictly to an aetiological or to an anatomical method of classification but are a mixture of both. The groups were chosen because they were found to be practical.

Patients who had more than one abnormality in their resected temporal lobe were placed in their relevant diagnostic groups and also categorized separately into a general group with the title 'Double pathology'.

The diagnostic headings were named as follows:
1. Developmental lesions
2. Trauma
3. Alien tissue
4. Ammon's horn sclerosis
5. Inflammatory
6. Indefinite
7. No apparent lesion
8. Double pathology

Group 1. Developmental lesions

Only those abnormalities widely regarded as developmental in origin were placed in this category. It is a heterogeneous collection and includes such conditions as arachnoid cysts, epidermoid cysts and heterotopic grey matter (Figs. 5, 6, 7).

Group 2. Trauma

This group contains all those patients whose temporal lobes show histological evidence of previous cerebral trauma. In most cases there was corroborative clinical evidence of a previous head injury. The essential histological feature is the presence of a focal scar and gliosis in the temporal cortex or white matter.

Group 3. Alien tissue

The main problems of classification were found in this category. The

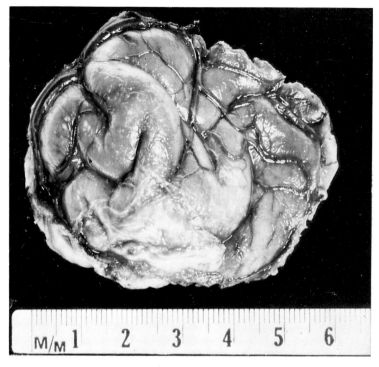

Fig. 5. Case 18. Lateral view of lobectomy specimen showing the whitish thickened leptomeninges of an arachnoid cyst.

criterion used for diagnosis was the presence within the lesion of abnormal or 'alien' nerve cells, glial cells, or other tissue elements.

Therefore all the cases which have been described previously as 'neoplasms', 'hamartomas', 'certain small tumours of the temporal lobe' (Cavanagh, 1958) and 'cortical dysplasia' (Taylor, Falconer, Bruton & Corsellis, 1971) are included irrespective of their suspected nature or origin. Within the context of the present study, which sets out to determine the nature, localization and development of different temporal lobe lesions, it seemed appropriate to avoid, in the initial stages at least, terms that already implied an origin or a mode of development. It also seemed appropriate to subdivide the Alien tissue group into categories based on the predominant variety of abnormal cell involved and for similar reasons the names of these categories were chosen to avoid the use of such terms as 'astrocytoma', 'oligodendroglioma' or 'angioma' which have a well-known and well-defined meaning. The three subdivisions were therefore selected in descriptive terms; cases fell readily into one of

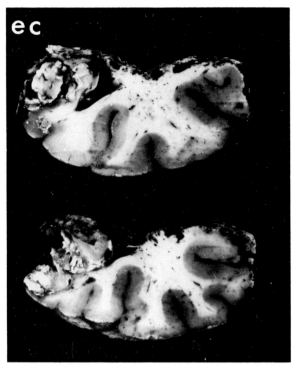

Fig. 6. Case 49. Keratin-filled epidermoid cyst (e.c.) lying medial to the inferior horn of the lateral ventricle.

these three groups: 3a. Glial lesion; 3b. Neuronoglial lesion; 3c. Vascular abnormality.

3a. Glial lesion

Three types of glial abnormality were defined by the predominant type of abnormal cell found in the lesion. Thus astrocytic glial lesions were composed of abnormal astrocytes (Fig. 8), oligodendrocytic glial lesions were composed of abnormal oligodendroglia (Figs. 9, 10) and mixed glial lesions contained both (Fig. 11).

3b. Neuronoglial lesion

The essential features in this subgroup were the presence of both abnormal nerve cells and abnormal glia within the same lesion. Two distinct and microscopically separate varieties of neuronoglial lesion became evident (Figs. 12, 13, 14). One corresponds to the cases of 'cortical dysplasia' (Taylor, Falconer, Bruton & Corsellis, 1971), the

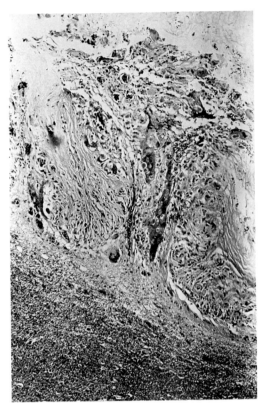

Fig. 7. Case 49. Epidermoid cyst. Cyst wall lined by squamous epithelial cells and the lumen filled with numerous layers of keratin. The white matter surrounding the cyst is intensely gliosed. (Haematoxylin & Eosin stain × 75)

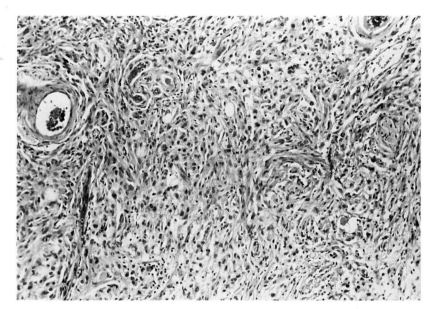

Fig. 8. Case 17. Astrocytic glial lesion composed mainly of spindle shaped fibrillary astrocytes which show some nuclear hyperchromasia (H & E × 125)

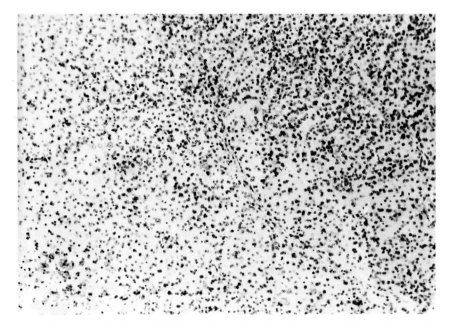

Fig. 9. Case 58. Amygdaloid nucleus showing clusters of hyperchromatic oligodendroglia partly replacing the normal amygdaloid architecture. (H & E × 125)

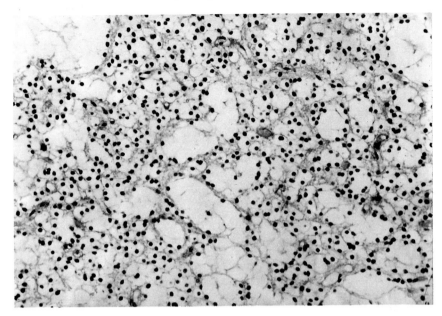

Fig. 10. Case 216. Oligodendroglial lesion replacing the normal white matter of the fusiform gyrus. The oligodendroglial cells have uniform hyperchromatic nuclei with their typical 'boxed nuclei' appearance. Numerous microcystic spaces are also visible. (H & E × 200)

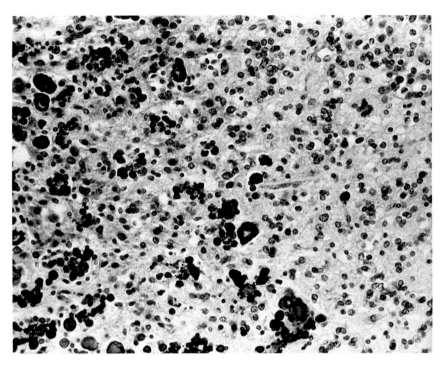

Fig. 11. Medium power view of a mixed glial lesion. Note the darkly stained calcospherites. The predominant cell in this area is a rather pleomorphic astrocyte. (H & E × 320)

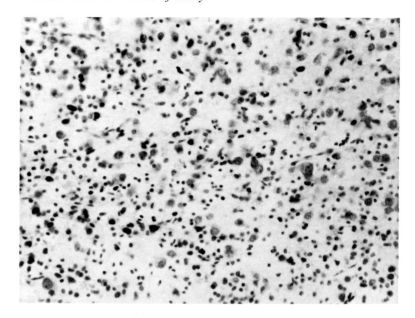

Fig. 12. Case 162. Ganglioglioma. Numerous large ganglion-like nerve cells are scattered haphazardly throughout the lesion. Abnormal astrocytes and oligo-dendroglia are also plentiful. (Van Gieson stain × 200)

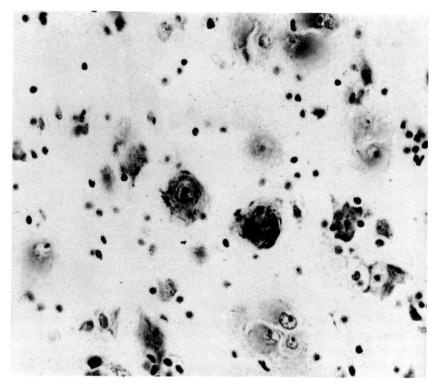

Fig. 13. Case 65. Cortical dysplasia showing giant nerve cells with plentiful deeply stained Nissl substance, large nuclei and crescentic thickening of the nuclear membrane. Abnormal glial cells are also visible. (Nissl × 320)

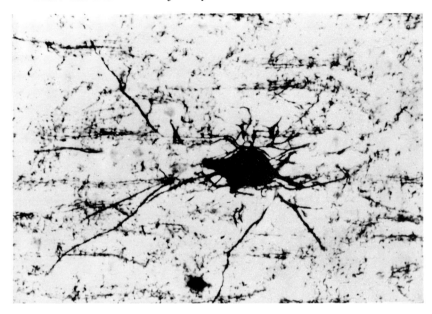

Fig. 14. Case 141. Cortical dysplasia. High power view of abnormal nerve cell showing the deep impregnation of neuronal processes with silver. (Gros. Biel. × 400)

other to the more commonly recognized entity of 'ganglioglioma' (Courville, 1930; Russell & Rubinstein, 1977).

3c.   *Vascular abnormality*

All cases placed into this category showed abnormal blood vessels or vascular spaces as the predominant histological feature (Figs. 15, 16).

Finally, the histological appearances of the Alien tissue group were assessed further in order to try to predict the eventual clinical outcome of the lobectomy. The following microscopic features were noted in each case:

    1. The presence of cellular pleomorphism.

    2. The presence of mitoses.

    3. The presence of calcification.

    4. Whether the lesion appeared to have been removed completely at operation.

Group 4.   Ammon's horn sclerosis

The temporal lobe damage seen in patients assigned to this group was originally called Ammon's horn sclerosis (Bouchet & Cazauvieilh, 1825;

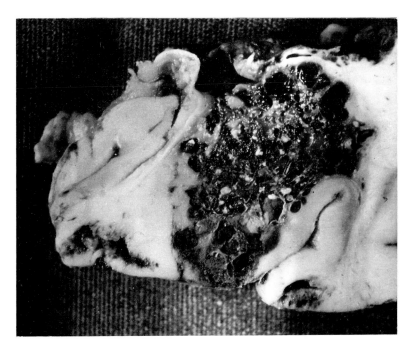

Fig. 15. Case 32. Coronal slice of surgical specimen showing a cavernous haemangioma. Note the honeycomb of thin-walled vascular spaces filled with blood. The anterior hippocampus is seen on the left.

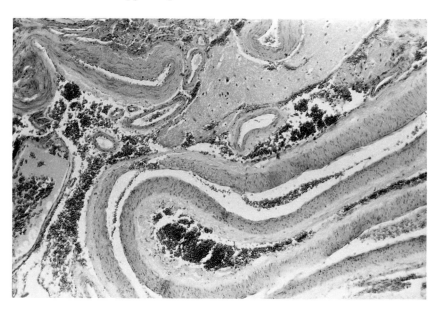

Fig. 16. Case 28. Medium power view of an arterio-venous vascular abnormality. The thin-walled venous space on the extreme left contrasts greatly with several thick-walled vessels at the top and on the right. (H & E × 28)

Sommer, 1880) but subsequent authors have preferred to use the names Incisural sclerosis (Earle, Baldwin & Penfield, 1953), Pararhinal sclerosis (Gastaut, 1959), Mesial temporal sclerosis (Falconer, Serafetinides & Corsellis, 1964) (Fig. 17a,b). Throughout the present study these terms have been used synonymously, although for historical reasons the term Ammon's horn sclerosis has been preferred. Nevertheless, it is realized that the less widely used and purely descriptive term of mesial temporal sclerosis is the more accurate anatomically as the sclerotic process often spreads beyond the confines of the Ammon's horn to involve other

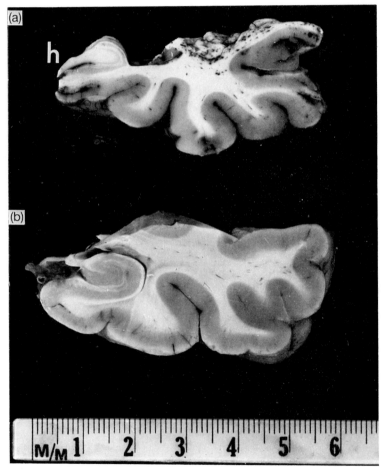

Fig. 17. a. Coronal slice from a temporal lobectomy specimen. The hippocampus (h) is whitish, shrunken, and shows almost total loss of the usual cortical architecture. b. A normal temporal lobe for comparison.

'mesial' temporal structures such as the parahippocampal gyrus, the amygdaloid nucleus, and the uncus.

Histologically the term Ammon's horn sclerosis denotes a patterned loss of nerve cells in the hippocampus which is accompanied by fibrous gliosis and eventually by shrinkage and atrophy (for normal picture see Fig. 18a). However, the nerve cell loss varies from case to case and three degrees of damage can be identified. In the commonest type the loss of hippocampal nerve cells is most severe and often almost total in two areas, the Sommer sector (H1) and the end folium (H3–5), less in the dentate fascia, and least in the resistant zone (H2) (Fig. 18b). This variety of lesion has been termed 'Classical' Ammon's horn sclerosis (Margerison & Corsellis, 1966). Other cases show an almost 'global' destruction of hippocampal neurons which I have described as 'Total' Ammon's horn sclerosis (Fig. 18c). Much less frequently the hippocampal nerve cell loss is minimal and involves only the end folium. Margerison and Corsellis (1966) called this 'end folium sclerosis' (Fig. 18d). In order to test the hypothesis that the severity of hippocampal damage might be related to the severity of the patient's epilepsy it seemed appropriate to subdivide all patients with Ammon's horn sclerosis into categories based on the degree of nerve cell loss. The subdivisions chosen correlate exactly with the three types of damage described above.

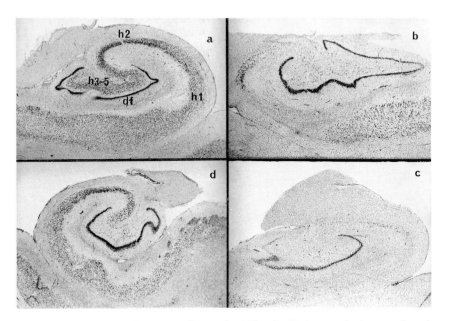

Fig. 18. a. Normal Ammon's horn. b. 'Classical' Ammon's horn sclerosis c. 'Total' Ammon's horn sclerosis. d. 'End folium sclerosis'. (Cresyl Violet × 6)

Group 5.   Inflammatory

This category contains all those cases which show microscopic evidence of inflammation whether or not the patient's clinical records produce corroborative evidence of past inflammatory illness. The histological damage varies in severity from widespread temporal lobe destruction compatible with an old necrotizing encephalitis or meningitis to a more circumscribed inflammatory focus representing the end result of a previous cerebral abscess (Figs. 19, 20).

Group 6.   Indefinite

The histological appearances of the lobes in this group were difficult to interpret. Indeed, the only reason for placing them together was the singular difficulty experienced by the examiner in determining whether the lobe was in fact abnormal. However, after careful examination it was

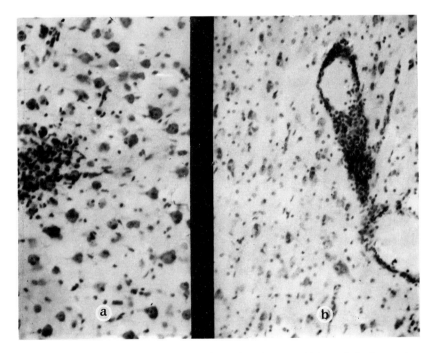

Fig. 19. Case 247. Medium power view showing a. glial nodule formation. b. perivascular cuffing, both typical features of a viral encephalitis. (Cresyl Violet × 200)

usually decided that the microscopic findings were on the borderline between the normal and abnormal lobe and the pathology was therefore described as 'Indefinite'. Some of the lobes show an unusual degree of gliosis without evidence of any neuronal loss either in the hippocampus, the amygdaloid nucleus, or the temporal lobe cortex. Others simply show an unexpected thickening of the leptomeninges or of the cerebral vessels (Fig. 21). In addition, a few cases have small numbers of unusually large neurons or a few large, bizarre glia scattered in the amygdaloid nucleus. Each of these subvarieties is discussed separately within the framework of the group as a whole.

Group 7.   No apparent lesion

This diagnostic category contains all the patients whose resected temporal lobe appeared normal on naked-eye examination.

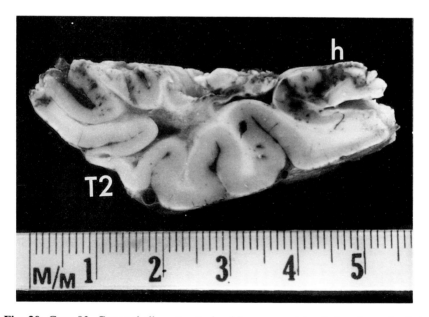

Fig. 20. Case 83. Coronal slice at anterior hippocampal level showing a healed abscess. In this block the middle temporal gyrus (T2) is most severely damaged and the cystic abscess cavity has destroyed the subjacent white matter. The anterior hippocampus (h) is seen on the right partly damaged by operative haemorrhage.

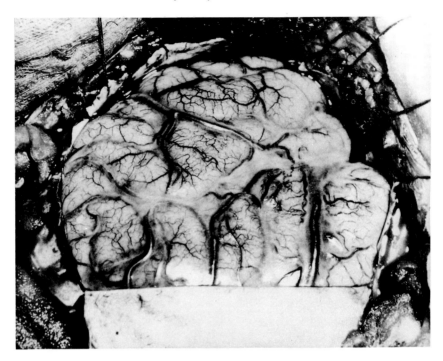

Fig. 21 Case 50. Operative photograph with the dura reflected downwards. In the depths of the sulcus which runs horizontally across the photograph the leptomeninges are thickened and opaque. Elsewhere the leptomeninges are intensely congested.

Group 8.   Double pathology

The final group contains all patients who had more than one histological abnormality in their resected lobe (Fig. 4). The cases were also included in the relevant diagnostic groups 1–7 above. In the vast majority of the patients one of the two lesions was an Ammon's horn sclerosis.

LOCALIZATION OF TEMPORAL LOBE ABNORMALITIES

After each case had been assigned to a diagnostic group the abnormalities were mapped out on a series of five line drawings representing five coronal slices cut at 1 cm level antero-posteriorly through the resected specimen. These coronal maps were labelled anatomically and thus a pictorial representation of each lesion was assembled. The maps were compiled from the photographic records, the naked-eye description of the lobe and the histological assessment of each specimen.

METHODOLOGICAL LIMITATIONS

Although the aim of the survey was to identify accurately the abnormalities found in a series of temporal lobe epileptic patients who had undergone anterior temporal lobectomy, the methods described above were subject to certain unavoidable limitations. These limitations were present in the initial choice of the sample of patients as well as in the collection of clinical and neuropathological data.

The sample

In some ways the sample of patients chosen for operation was not typical of those with temporal lobe epilepsy as a whole in that it included only the most severely affected patients whose seizures were frequent and poorly controlled by anticonvulsant medication. Therefore it has not been suggested that the nature or relative incidence of abnormalities in the present study is identical to that which might be found in another group of temporal lobe epileptics in whom the fits are well controlled by drugs.

Clinical data

Clinical information was obtained from the patient's records. Some clinical notes were incomplete in that the information was not known or had been forgotten by the informant. Similarly, some patients did not attend for follow-up, a few lived overseas, and others changed their address and became untraceable. In addition, an objective assessment of the success or failure of the lobectomy was not always easy. First, the length of follow-up varied from case to case: the most recent operations had very little follow-up information on which to base an accurate assessment. Secondly, there were a few borderline cases where the success or failure of the operation was difficult to establish. Nevertheless these judgements were made by the author and not by a member of the neurosurgical team; to this extent they are hoped to be free from bias.

Neuropathology

Not all the temporal lobes were photographed and some of the early specimens were described in an unformalized fashion. Therefore in certain cases the accurate localization of temporal lobe damage was difficult. In addition, the exact extent of the surgical ablation varied from case to case; the more medial structures such as the hippocampus and the amygdaloid nucleus were destroyed occasionally by the surgeon's sucker. This could lead to difficulty in diagnosis, a fact which is reflected and discussed in the neuropathological findings.

Finally, a review of the histological material necessitated an examination of tissue sections which may have been stored for more than 25 years. Some deterioration of the slides had occurred and made diagnosis difficult. This was most marked in a small group of cases which were mounted in an experimental plastic mounting medium instead of canada balsam or one of the more modern resin mixtures (for example, the resin mixture known as XAM).

3. Results and discussion

The usefulness of an investigation depends on the conclusions which can be drawn from an examination of the relevant data. In the present survey, an analysis of the information has highlighted certain differences between the diagnostic groups, not only with respect to the clinical presentation and behaviour but also in the long term effects of surgery. These differences are discussed in the order given below. Nevertheless, in order to avoid a tedious catalogue of data, the results from which the conclusions are drawn are presented in tabular form as an appendix at the end of Chapter 4. A brief summary of the case histories is also included in the appendix. The coded case numbers which identify each patient are used throughout the text.

1. **Clinical features**
    (a) Influence of age.
    (b) Influence of sex.
    (c) Side of lobectomy.
    (d) Possible predisposing factors.
        (i)   Birth injury.
        (ii) Head injury.
        (iii) Febrile convulsions in infancy.
        (iv) Status epilepticus.
    (e) The effects of operation.
        (i)   Post-operative complications.
        (ii) Death rate and cause of death.
        (iii) Effect of lobectomy on fit frequency.
        (iv) Effect of lobectomy on psychiatric illness, personality, and social adjustment.
2. **Neuropathological features**
    (a) Classification and diagnosis.
    (b) Diagnostic difficulties.
        (i)   Defects of tissue processing and staining.
        (ii) Problems of anatomy: site of lesion.
        (iii) Problems of anatomy: extent of surgical resection.
        (iv) Errors of diagnosis.
    (c) Diagnostic groups.
        1. Developmental abnormalities.
        2. Trauma.
        3. Alien tissue lesions.

        3(a) Glial lesions.
              (i)   Astrocytic glial lesions.
              (ii) Oligodendrocytic glial lesions.
              (iii) Mixed glial lesions.
        3(b) Neuronoglial lesions.
              (i)   Ganglioglial lesions.
              (ii) Cortical dysplasia.
        3(c) Vascular abnormalities.
    4.   Ammon's horn sclerosis.
    5.   Inflammatory lesion.
    6.   Indefinite pathology.
    7.   No apparent abnormality.
    8.   Double pathology.

1. CLINICAL FEATURES

(a) Influence of age

In patients with temporal lobe epilepsy the onset of the disorder is usually timed from the age at first seizure. However, some writers consider it to be the age at which the patient experienced his or her first attack of 'chronic epilepsy' (Jensen, 1976b). Because of this the comparison of results is difficult to assess. Nevertheless the study of age factors in the present report has produced a number of interesting observations (Tables 1, 2, 3, 4).

The mean age at first epileptic fit (10.6 years) and at operation (20.06 years) compares closely with many of the surgical reports (Jensen,

Table 1. *Age variation with neuropathological diagnosis*

Diagnostic group	No. of cases in group	Mean age at first fit (yrs)	Mean age at operation (yrs)
Ammon's horn sclerosis	107	5.19	22.64
Inflammatory	8	8.62	24.75
Double pathology	18	9.53	22.33
Indefinite	25	14.72	31.24
No apparent lesion	41	15.37	28.56
Alien tissue lesion	38	16.93	26.77
Trauma	7	17.31	33.14
Developmental lesion	5	22.80	38.20

Table 2. *Age at first fit/age at operation: difference between Ammon's horn sclerotics and other diagnostic categories*

Diagnostic groups compared with Ammon's horn sclerotics	Age at first fit Difference between the two means	Age at operation Difference between the two means
Inflammatory	$P < 0.1$	$P < 0.5$
Double pathology	$P < 0.05$	$P < 0.5$
Indefinite	$P < 0.0001$	$P < 0.0001$
No apparent lesion	$P < 0.0001$	$P < 0.002$
Alien tissue lesion	$P < 0.0001$	$P < 0.01$
Trauma	$P < 0.01$	$P < 0.02$
Developmental lesion	$P < 0.01$	$P < 0.0001$

Table 3. *Age variation within Alien tissue lesions*

Alien tissue subgroups	No. of cases in subgroup	Mean age at first fit (yrs)	Mean age at operation (yrs)
Neuronoglial:			
(Ganglioglial)	5	6.44	17.60
Mixed glial	9	11.11	19.67
Neuronoglial:			
(Cortical dysplasia)	8	14.75	26.88
Vascular	3	16.00	23.66
Oligodendrocytic glial	5	26.00	38.20
Astrocytic glial	8	27.25	34.63

Table 4. *Age at first fit and age at operation: difference between ganglioglial and other subgroups*

Subgroups compared with ganglioglial lesions	Age at first fit Difference between the two means	Age at operation Difference between the two means
Mixed glial	$P < 0.2$	$P < 0.5$
Cortical dysplasia	$P < 0.05$	$P < 0.1$
Vascular	$P < 0.1$	$P < 0.5$
Oligodendrocytic glial	$P < 0.01$	$P < 0.005$
Astrocytic glial	$P < 0.002$	$P < 0.01$

1976b). Females have a slightly younger age at onset than males but the difference is not significant.

More important, however, the sample shows several clearly defined and statistically significant differences between the age at first fit and the various pathological categories. These differences may provide a basis for subsequent identification and selection of patients for operation.

Thus epilepsy tends to begin earliest in those patients with Ammon's horn sclerosis (mean age 5.19 years), the largest single diagnostic group. The early age at first fit in these patients may relate to their close association with febrile convulsions which are known to occur almost entirely in children under five years old (Millichap, 1968).

The inflammatory group also shows a young age at first fit (mean age 8.62 years, $P < 0.1$) probably reflecting the higher incidence of cerebral infection in young children (*Registrar General's Statistical Review of England and Wales*, 1972). In contrast, and quite unexpectedly, the five patients with 'developmental' lesions had the latest age onset (mean age 22.8 years, $P < 0.01$). Logically one would have expected a 'developmental' lesion to give rise to symptoms early in life and indeed the massive series of 'organic' epilepsy compiled by Lennox & Lennox (1960) showed that 44 per cent had their first fit under five years of age. However, the small number of patients in the developmental group may make the present figures rather artificial.

Within the Alien tissue group there were further statistically significant variations when the age at first fit was compared with the histological variety of the lesion.

Thus the ganglioglial lesions and mixed glial lesions (mean age at first fit 6.44 years and 11.11 years respectively) differ markedly in age at first fit from the astrocytic and oligodendrocytic subgroups (mean age 26.00 years and 27.25 years), a fact which supports the suggestion that these subgroups may have a different aetiology.

The remaining diagnostic categories had an average age onset of epilepsy between 14 and 17 years which is the usual peak incidence for temporal lobe epilepsy (Lennox & Lennox, 1960).

The mean age at operation in the diagnostic groups followed closely the variations in the age at first fit although it was, in general, some 15 years later. Thus there was no evidence that any particular group was operated upon at an earlier age than any other and in this respect it must be assumed that no one type of temporal lobe lesion produced a more disabling type of temporal lobe fit.

(b)   Influence of sex

The incidence of cryptogenic and of temporal lobe epilepsy is usually higher in men (Lennox & Lennox, 1960, p. 502), but the numerical inequality between the sexes is not normally great. One example quoted by Lennox & Lennox is the 53-year review of patients' records at the Craig epileptic colony where male epileptics formed 51.1 per cent of the total.

However, in Jensen's temporal lobe surgery material the male/female ratio was as high as 1.39/1 (Jensen, 1976a), and in the present series it is even higher (male/female ratio 1.7/1, $P < 0.0001$), although an adequate explanation for these figures is difficult to find. Certainly a preponderance of males might have been expected in some diagnostic groups, for febrile convulsions, head injuries and developmental cerebral abnormalities are all more common in boys than girls (Lennox & Lennox, 1960; Taylor, 1969b). However, in the other neuropathological categories the reasons are unclear.

One possible explanation may be the effect on behaviour of the temporal lobe fits which in males tend to be more violent and socially disruptive, thus producing a greater demand for treatment. A second factor may be the relatively higher incidence of psychosis in female temporal lobe epileptics (Taylor, 1971) which would tend to exclude more females in the pre-operative selection process.

On the other hand there may be some sex-linked susceptibility to temporal lobe seizures in boys. A full review of the fascinating problem of the sexual differences in disease has been undertaken by Taylor (1981b) using much of the material from his studies of epilepsy, and although many questions could not be answered, he showed clearly the profound and complex influence of gender in many types of illness, including temporal lobe fits.

(c) Side of lobectomy

Taylor (1969b and 1981b) has also investigated the possible relationships between the side of lobectomy, the sex of the patient and the age at first fit. The present series contained almost equal numbers of right and left-sided operations (Table 5). There was only one bilateral operation (Case No. 179), performed on a man who had a second temporal lobe removed some two years after the first. The second post-operative course was disastrous, ending with death in uncontrolled status epilepticus one year afterwards. No further bilateral operations were performed, especially as the results of other unsuccessful bilateral operations were beginning to be published (Scoville, Dunsmore, Liberson, Henry & Pepe, 1953; Scoville & Milner, 1957).

Table 5. *Variation with sex and age*

Variation with sex of the patient

Left lobectomy:	80 men 47 women	M/F ratio 1.7:1
Right lobectomy:	75 men 46 women	M/F ratio 1.63:1

Variation with age at first fit and age at operation

Right lobectomy:	Mean age at first fit 10.97 years (S.D. 11.38)
	Mean age at operation 26.21 years (S.D. 10.78)
Left lobectomy:	Mean age at first fit 10.80 years (S.D. 12.12)
	Mean age at operation 25.93 years (S.D. 11.55)

(d) Possible predisposing factors

(i) Birth injury

The relationship of birth injury to temporal lobe epilepsy has been a matter of debate since the results of Earle, Baldwin, & Penfield's study were published in 1953. They examined 157 patients who had had a temporal lobectomy and claimed to have found macroscopic pathological changes in every lobe; of these no less than 100 patients showed damage which suggested compression or anoxia of the brain at birth or in early infancy. The pathological changes varied from atrophy or toughness of a single gyrus to more extensive atrophy involving almost the whole lobe. The authors advanced the hypothesis that such changes resulted from incisural herniation of the medial temporal lobe through the tentorium cerebelli during a difficult or protracted birth leading to ischaemia of the nervous tissue via compression of the adjacent posterior cerebral and anterior choroidal arteries. Later the resulting scarred tissue 'ripened' into an epileptogenic focus. It is interesting to note that only 10 per cent of their series had a documented history of difficult birth.

The theory of 'incisural sclerosis' was questioned by Meyer, Falconer, and Beck (1954), who stated that if 'distortion of the head during parturition is the crucial factor, a history of difficult birth in patients with mesial temporal sclerosis should be particularly common'. In addition, they quoted Norman (1963), who remarked that occlusion of the posterior cerebral and anterior choroidal artery usually leads to damage of the pallidum and this area is almost invariably spared in epilepsy. Nevertheless Falconer, Serafetinides, and Corsellis (1964) did find a history of difficult birth in 13 of their 47 cases but, although high, this latter figure was not significant. Similarly, Ounsted, Lindsay, and Norman (1966) found that birth injury was not of statistical significance in the causation of temporal lobe epilepsy.

The findings from the present study go some way to reconcile the disparate views expressed previously. Thirty-two patients (13 per cent of the total) were reported to have suffered some degree of birth injury. Of these patients, 20 proved to have had an Ammon's horn sclerosis (Table 6). The figures show that birth injury is a significant predisposing factor in the Ammon's horn sclerotic group at the level of $P < 0.02$. In summary, therefore, a history of birth trauma does seem to contribute to the development of some cases of Ammon's horn sclerosis. The exact mechanism, however, must remain in doubt.

(ii) Head injury

On the other hand, there is no disputing the importance of head injury in the subsequent development of fits. About 40 per cent of all patients who sustain an 'open' head injury become epileptic within five years (Russell & Whitty, 1952). The figure for 'closed' head injuries is less, but still approaches 10 per cent (Jennett, 1965). Scarring may occur in any area of brain which is injured and the temporal lobes are known to be very commonly affected in cerebral trauma (Strich, 1976).

For the purposes of the present review, the diagnosis of cerebral trauma was made by neuropathological observation and was not based on a history of previous head injury. Thus, only those patients whose resected temporal lobe showed definite evidence of a cortical or white matter scar were assigned to the Trauma group. The area of brain immediately surrounding a cortical scar is always more heavily gliosed than normal, but cases where the resected temporal lobe showed only a heavy gliosis without definite scar formation were excluded. Indeed, the cases which showed only an excessive gliosis were placed in the Indefinite pathology category.

Some degree of head injury had been noted in thirty-eight patients (15 per cent) of the present series (see Table 6). This included six of the seven patients assigned to the Trauma group, seven of the twenty-five patients with Indefinite pathology and 11 of the 107 with Ammon's horn sclerosis. From these figures it is seen that a clinical history of previous head injury is, as expected, a highly significant predisposing factor in the Trauma group ($P < 0.0001$). It is also significant in the Indefinite pathology group at the level of $P < 0.01$. These latter figures suggest that some Indefinite pathology lesions may have been produced by 'trauma'.

(iii) Febrile convulsions

Febrile convulsions are nowadays a well-known factor in the pathogenesis of temporal lobe epilepsy, especially where the resected lobe contained a sclerotic Ammon's horn (Falconer, Serafetinides & Corsellis, 1964; Ounsted, Lindsay & Norman, 1966; Falconer & Taylor, 1968). Fifty-five patients (22 per cent of the present series) had a history of febrile convulsions in infancy and no less than 50 of these were found to have a sclerotic Ammon's horn (see Table 6). This correlates with the Ammon's horn sclerosis group at the level of $P < 0.0001$. The exact mechanisms producing the damage, however, are not nearly so clear-cut. Meldrum (1983) and Corsellis and Meldrum (1984) have summarized previous theories based on information from human and animal research. Meldrum (1983) has produced a 'revised metabolic hypothesis for epileptic brain damage' which stresses the 'primary role of enhanced energy demand during seizure activity (i.e. consumptive hypoxia) with a possible secondary role for relative insufficiency of substrate delivery (due to local impairment of blood flow, arterial hypotension and other systemic changes)'. Damage occurred in selectively vulnerable neurons which appear to have a greater tendency to show 'bursting activity' and a 'paroxysmal depolarizing shift' associated with enhanced calcium ion entry.

Thus Meldrum, by using modern, experimental methods, brings together to some degree the earlier hypotheses of Vogt and Vogt (1922), Spielmeyer (1927), and also of Scholz (1933).

(iv) Status epilepticus

The influence of status epilepticus in the pathogenesis of temporal lobe and cryptogenic epilepsy has been studied by various workers (Cavanagh & Meyer, 1956; Norman, 1964; Falconer, Serafetinides & Corsellis, 1964; Ounsted, Lindsay & Norman, 1966; Margerison & Corsellis, 1966; Corsellis & Meldrum, 1984), notwithstanding the fact that a precise clinical definition of status epilepticus is often difficult and also the fact that some episodes of status epilepticus may not be recorded in the patient's notes. Nevertheless, Cavanagh and Meyer (1956) found a 64 per cent incidence of status epilepticus in a group of 17 patients with Ammon's horn sclerosis and no history of status epilepticus in a group of nine patients without the lesion.

The present survey found that 25 patients had had one or more recorded episodes of status epilepticus before lobectomy. Sixteen of these patients had a sclerotic Ammon's horn; a significant association with the Ammon's horn sclerosis group at the level of $P < 0.02$ (see Table 6).

However, the picture becomes more complex when it is realized that severe febrile convulsions can often culminate in an episode of status epilepticus and no less than 12 of the 16 Ammon's horn sclerotic patients with a history of status epilepticus also had a recorded history of febrile convulsions in infancy.

Thus, though a bout of status epilepticus may be a predisposing factor in certain cases of Ammon's horn sclerosis, it seems no more likely to be so than an episode of febrile convulsions in infancy. Indeed, the critical factor is probably the age of the victim rather than the severity of the fit,

Table 6. *Variation of predisposing factors with neuropathological diagnosis*

Predisposing Factors	Neuropathological groups and number of patients in group								
	Developmental (5 cases)	Trauma (7 cases)	Alien tissue (38 cases)	AHS (107 cases)	Inflammatory (8 cases)	Indefinite (25 cases)	No apparent lesion (41 cases)	Double pathology (18 cases)	Total No. of cases
Birth injury	0	1	2	20	0	2	4	3	32
Febrile convulsions	0	0	0	50	1	2	1	1	55
Status epilepticus	0	0	0	16	0	1	4	4	25
Head injury	1	6	3	11	2	7	5	3	38

for fatal status epilepticus, when it occurs in children, nearly always produces massive acute brain damage, but is much less commonly associated with such damage in adults (Corsellis & Bruton, 1983).

(e) The effects of operation

(i) Post-operative complications

Jensen (1975a) analysed the published data from fifteen separate temporal lobectomy studies involving a total of 858 patients. The most serious post-operative complication was a permanent hemiplegia (2.45 per cent), whilst another 4.2 per cent had a temporary hemiparesis. Aphasia occurred in 5.2 per cent of patients but this often improved with speech therapy. Only Maspes and Marossero (1953) claimed a trouble-free post-operative course in their series of 28 patients. In the present study only nine patients (3.6 per cent) had significant post-operative complications (Table 7). Six of the nine were left with a permanent hemiparesis, one was dysphasic, another ataxic, and the last exhibited unusual athetoid movements. It should be noted that six of the nine affected patients were operated upon before 1956 in the early years when the technique was being refined. This coincides with Jensen's conclusions that the chances of severe post-operative complications have decreased markedly over the years and are now very uncommon.

(ii) Death rate and cause of death

Post-operative fatalities. Jensen's (1975a) review of the literature also showed a death rate of 7.9 per 1000 lobectomies in the immediate post-

Table 7.   *Post-operative complications*

Case No.	Post-operative disability	Diagnostic category
16	Hemiplegia	Inflammatory
51	Hemiplegia	No abnormality
71	Hemiplegia	Ammon's horn sclerosis
72	Hemiplegia	Astrocytic glial lesion
176	Hemiplegia	Ammon's horn sclerosis
238	Hemiplegia	Neuronoglial lesion
30	Dysphasia	Vascular
48	Athetotic movements	Inflammatory
231	Ataxia	No abnormality

operative period, most deaths occurring in the early years during the development of the operation. These deaths resulted from a mixture of pulmonary, cardiac, or cerebral events; pulmonary complications were most common. In the present study no patient died as a direct result of surgery, an undoubted tribute to the skill of the neurosurgeon and his team.

Long-term death rate. An analysis of the long-term death rate, however, has proved to be more complex. Tables 8 and 9 show that a total of 27 patients in the present series are known to have died in the 25-year follow-up period. This represents a total of 108 deaths per thousand lobectomies, which is about double the recorded rate of non-operated epileptics (Pond, Bidwell & Stein, 1960; Henriksen, Juul-Jensen & Lund, 1970) and about eight times the average death rate from all causes in England and Wales (*Registrar General's Statistical Review for England and Wales*, 1972). The figure is also double the average rate reported by Jensen (1975b) who found a total of 47.6 deaths per thousand temporal lobectomies. Jensen had, however, excluded all those who had died in the immediate post-operative period and all those who had died as a result of a recurrence of a temporal lobe tumour which had been found at lobectomy. When the same criteria are applied in the present series, the death rate is reduced by 20 per cent. Furthermore, the follow-up period of the present study covered a time span of twenty-five years, by which time a number of patients had died from causes unrelated to their operation. Removal of these patients reduced the death rate even further. Notwithstanding these statistical complexities the data from all studies suggests that the death rate after temporal lobectomy is not much greater

Table 8. *Post-operative deaths*

Cause of death	No. of cases	M/F ratio	% of total sample	Average survival time after operation
Epilepsy	10	10/0	4.0	3.4 yrs
Recurrence of lesion	5	3/2	2.0	10.4 yrs
Suicide	6	4/2	2.4	5.6 yrs
Unrelated cause	6	5/1	2.4	10.0 yrs

Total No. of deaths 27 (11% of sample).
Male/Female ratio 4.4/1.
Average survival time after lobectomy (all causes) 7.2 yrs.

Table 9. *Death following operation: cause of death and length of survival*

Case No.	Cause of death	Diagnostic category	Sex	Age at operation (yrs)	Survival after operation (yrs)
29	Epileptic fit	Ammon's horn sclerosis	M	20	5
50	Status epilepticus	Equivocal	M	21	6
110	Status epilepticus	Ammon's horn sclerosis	M	33	1
117	Epileptic fit	Trauma	M	17	1
130	Epileptic fit	Inflammatory	M	10	3
143	Epileptic fit	Ammon's horn sclerosis	M	20	4
169	Status epilepticus	Equivocal	M	16	8
179	Status epilepticus	No abnormality found	M	25 27 }	3
185	Status epilepticus	No abnormality found	M	17	3
212	Epileptic fit	No abnormality found	M	41	4 months
49	Recurrence of lesion	Developmental abnormality	M	36	7
72	Recurrence of lesion	Astrocytic glial lesion	F	35	8
103	Recurrence of lesion	Oligodendrocytic glial lesion	F	51	15
194	Recurrence of lesion	Astrocytic glial lesion	M	55	2
235	Recurrence of lesion	Oligodendrocytic glial lesion	M	56	20

32	Suicide	Vascular lesion	M	19	2
138	Suicide	No abnormality found	M	42	1
139	Suicide	Ammon's horn sclerosis	F	26	6
144	Suicide	Neuronoglial lesion	M	16	14
206	Suicide	Ammon's horn sclerosis	F	16	9
221	Suicide	Equivocal	M	34	2
76	Unrelated cause	Trauma	M	45	17
91	Unrelated cause	Mixed glial lesion	M	38	1
118	Unrelated cause	No abnormality found	F	14	Unknown
141	Unrelated cause	Neuronoglial lesion	M	46	15
162	Unrelated cause	Neuronoglial lesion	M	23	15
176	Cause unknown	Ammon's horn sclerosis	M	16	2

than the expected rate in non-operated epileptics and when it is remembered that lobectomy patients are drawn from the most severely handicapped cases, it becomes manifest that the operation is a remarkably safe procedure.

Cause of death. An examination of the mode of death shows definite similarities between lobectomy patients and non-operated epileptics (Henriksen, Juul-Jensen & Lund, 1970). In the present study, 37 per cent of deaths occurred in an epileptic fit or related to a bout of status epilepticus (see Tables 8 and 9). (The Danish figures were 26 per cent.) Deaths from suicide in the present study were as high as 22 per cent: similarly, the Danish workers found no less than 20 per cent of their series committed suicide. In addition, Henriksen, Juul-Jensen, and Lund (1970) noted that a further 11 per cent of their patients died as a result of 'an accident'. Bearing in mind the difficulties of determining an accurate cause in some cases where death is sudden and unexpected, I found that the figures from both series show definite associations.

Taylor and Marsh (1977) have also reviewed the causes of death in temporal lobectomy patients, and in a personal communication in 1982 Taylor emphasized the problem of finding an accurate cause of death by quoting a case from the present study which presented at the Coroner's court. The patient was found drowned in a canal and the Coroner's verdict was suicide; this verdict has been used by the present author. However, Taylor noted that 'the patient had his teeth in his pocket'. Apparently he always put his teeth in his pocket when he was about to have a fit. Thus, Taylor felt that the death might have occurred in an epileptic convulsion rather than as the result of a suicide attempt.

Despite these problems of classification, the figures show that no less than 60 per cent of deaths in the present series were sudden and unexpected, a fact which highlights the essentially capricious nature of the disease. The corresponding figures from Henriksen, Juul-Jensen, and Lund's 1970 study of non-operated epileptics were 57 per cent, which suggests that the operation itself does not alter adversely the natural course of the epileptic process.

(iii) Effects of lobectomy on fit frequency

The question in the mind of an epileptic person or his family when offered a temporal lobectomy, however, is unlikely to be whether the operation will alter adversely the natural course of his epileptic process. They are more likely to ask simply whether the operation will cure the fits and, in this context, the neurosurgical team at the Guy's, Maudsley Hospital Neurosurgical Unit began actively to determine an answer as soon as the first patient attended for follow-up. The results of their continuing studies have been published over the years (Hill, Pond, Mitchell & Falconer, 1957; Falconer & Serafetinides, 1963; Falconer, Serafetinides & Corsellis, 1964; Taylor & Falconer, 1968).

Falconer, Serafetinides, and Corsellis (1964), studied 100 consecutive lobectomies and compared the clinical results with the neuropathological findings. They found that the results were best whenever the excised specimen contained a definite lesion. However, they found also that some patients without a definite lesion had benefited from surgery, while, conversely, a few patients with lesions had not. Finally, they stressed the need for further post-mortem studies to provide more accurate information. As already quoted, Jensen (1976b) supplemented the previous study with a comprehensive review of the world literature. She divided the results into six groups based on an original assessment procedure designed by Penfield and Steelman (1947) in which patients were interviewed and assessed for the preceding twelve months. Groups I and II were successful operations, Group III was a worthwhile operation, Groups IV and V were unsuccessful and Group VI had no follow-up. Jensen observed a wide scatter of results, especially in those patients who became fit-free. The percentage of fit-free patients varied from 28 to 62 per cent according to the survey involved. She concluded that the major factor contributing to the widely scattered results was the anatomical extent of the operation. Thus, those operations in which the resection included the uncus, the parahippocampal gyrus, the hippocampus, and the amygdaloid nucleus had produced the best results. On average, Jensen found that 43 per cent were fit-free and another 18 per cent had a marked reduction in their fits, a total of almost two-thirds having been improved by operation.

Jensen and Klinken (1976) took the survey further when they compared the clinical results with the neuropathological findings when these were available. They agreed with Falconer, Serafetinides, and Corsellis (1964) who had concluded that the best results occurred in those cases where the neuropathological abnormality was definite and appeared to be circumscribed.

The Danish results were complicated, however, not only by the variety of surgical operation but also by the limitation to a one-year assessment. Epileptic fits can occur at very infrequent intervals and it would be unwise to call a patient 'fit-free' if he has not had a fit in the preceding twelve months. Nevertheless, the data provide an important comparison with the present research in which all temporal lobes were removed in a standardized *en bloc* fashion and in which the average length of follow-up for 94 per cent of the 249 patients was more than eight years.

In the present study the term 'fit-free' has not been used. Patients were classed as Greatly improved, Improved, Unaltered, or Worse. They were placed in the Greatly improved category only if they had been free of fits for at least five years, and thus, by definition, no patient who had been followed up for less than five years could be classed as Greatly improved even if he had been free from convulsions since operation. The group of Improved patients contains all those who had been fit-free for less than

Table 10. *Long-term results of surgery: 234 patients by diagnostic category*

Group	Total No. of cases in each group	Effect on fits				Effect on personality and/or social adjustment				
		Greatly improved	Improved	Unaltered	Worse	Greatly improved	Improved	Unaltered	Worse	No F/U
Developmental lesion	(5)	1	1	2	1	1	1	1	2	(0)
Trauma	(7)	2	1	3	1	0	0	6	1	(0)
Alien tissue										
Astrocytic	(8)	3	3	0	2	4	2	2	0	(0)
Oligodendrocytic	(5)	1	2	0	2	0	2	3	0	(0)
Mixed glial	(9)	5	3	0	1	5	2	0	2	(0)
Neuronoglial (ganglioglial)	(5)	3	1	0	1	1	1	0	3	(0)
Neuronoglial (cortical dysplasia)	(8)	1	5	2	0	1	4	3	0	(0)
Vascular	(3)	0	3	0	0	0	1	1	1	(0)
Ammon's horn sclerosis	(107)	37	43	13	7	34	30	26	10	(7)
Inflammatory	(8)	0	5	2	0	0	3	3	1	(1)
Indefinite	(25)	5	3	8	6	3	2	10	7	(3)
No apparent abnormality	(41)	8	9	7	14	4	4	13	17	(3)
Double pathology	(18)	8	6	1	2	5	2	5	5	(1)

Total No. of sample 249
No F/U information 15

Post-operative sample 234

five years and those whose fits had been reduced substantially. In all, 68 per cent were Greatly improved or Improved, and 32 per cent were Unaltered or Worse, a statistically significant degree of improvement after operation at the level of $P < 0.001$.

An analysis of the data by diagnostic group (Tables 10 and 11a, b) reveals that most of the improvement is confined to two diagnostic categories. Thus in the Ammon's horn sclerotic group 80 patients were Greatly improved or Improved, with 20 patients Unaltered or Worse ($P < 0.05$). Further analysis showed that the improvement in the Alien tissue group was confined to the mixed glial and the ganglioglial subgroups where the chance of being improved was significant at the levels $P < 0.005$ and $P < 0.05$ respectively. The remaining groups showed no significant alteration in fit pattern after operation.

It appears, therefore, that the effects of lobectomy on fit frequency do vary with the type of pathology in the resected lobe and that certain groups with circumscribed specific neuropathology benefit considerably more than others. These factors are discussed more fully in the section on neuropathological diagnosis.

Table 11a. *Results of surgery on epileptic fits*
234 cases with F/U information

Greatly improved	Improved	Unaltered	Worse
76	84	38	36

Greatly improved and improved	160 (68%)
Unaltered or worse	74 (32%)

Table 11b. *Results of surgery on personality and social adjustment*
234 cases with F/U information

Greatly improved	Improved	Unaltered	Worse
59	53	73	49

Greatly improved and improved	112 (48%)
Unaltered or worse	122 (52%)

(iv) Effects of lobectomy on psychiatric illness, personality, and social adjustment

Psychiatric disturbances in epilepsy are common and have excited comment in many classical studies (Esquirol, 1838; Falret, 1860; Hughlings Jackson, 1875; Gowers, 1901; Turner W. A., 1907). However, current knowledge of the interrelationships between personality change, depression, psychosis, and epilepsy still remains slender (Trimble, 1981). Nevertheless, the operation of temporal lobectomy provides a unique opportunity to analyse any such relationships as may exist between mental symptoms and certain brain lesions even though the analyses are likely to be glib and misleading (Taylor, 1981a). With this in mind, temporal lobectomy should not be judged solely by its effect on fit frequency; there must be some attempt to study the effect on the patient's ability to live a 'normal independent life', as this is at least as important as a reduction in the number of fits. Jensen (1976c) attempted such a study by comparing the effects of operation on the patient's subsequent social and psychiatric status. She found that the relief of seizures was the most important factor in obtaining 'a normal working capacity' but that the psychological status of people with few or no fits determined to a large extent their degree of independence.

In the present review, an attempt was made to glean information on the subsequent work record, home life, marriage, and so forth, as well as the mental state, and to compare this with the pre-operative data. In addition, special attention was paid to three overtly psychiatric features; depression, aggression, and schizophrenia, as these were considered to be particularly relevant indices of normal social integration. However, the assessment of a 'normal independent life' is much more subjective than the enumeration of the daily number of fits, especially when the only information available is the patient's medical records. Nevertheless, importance was placed on such items as a return to full-time work, subsequent marriage, mixing socially, living away from institutional care, and so forth, as a general index of normality. Patients were classed as Greatly improved, Improved, Unaltered, or Worse, using the same categories as were chosen for the measurements of effect on fit frequency. There is no denying that the assessments were in some cases more difficult to make than those on fit pattern but after reading the detailed follow-up material which covered a period of 10–15 years it was often surprisingly easy to arrive at a justifiable conclusion.

The results of the study are given in Tables 10 to 14, and show that in the whole group, lobectomy produces no significant alteration in personality and social adjustment, but when the results are analysed by diagnostic categories (see Table 10) certain significant changes are seen. Thus, the Ammon's horn sclerotic group has a highly significant chance of being improved ($P < 0.001$) in contrast to the Trauma group, the

Indefinite pathology group, and the No apparent abnormality group, whose members are significantly worse after operation ($P < 0.05$, $P < 0.01$, and $P < 0.005$ respectively). In the other diagnostic categories, personality and social adjustment are not altered significantly.

Armed with this information, one may compare the effects of operation on psychosocial adjustment with the results of operation on fit frequency to produce a 'league table' of benefit from operation. This is discussed later.

Incidence of depression. Griesinger (1857) commented that a misanthropic perversion of sentiment, sometimes with actual melancholia and suicidal tendency, was observed in a great many epileptic patients. Other authors have confirmed his views (Williams, 1956; Henriksen, Juul-Jensen & Lund, 1970), yet Pond (1957) found fewer than a dozen suicides in a series of many hundreds of epileptic patients and considered that suicide was quite rare. In the present study only one patient (0.4 per cent) was considered depressed at the time of operation; afterwards the incidence of depression rose to 10 per cent ($P < 0.0001$) (Table 12) and during the follow-up period six patients committed suicide. These figures represent a highly significant rise in the rate of depression after operation, the mechanisms of which are obscure. However, it is known that the incidence of depression is much higher in temporal lobe epilepsy than in other varieties of the disease (Barraclough, 1981). Weil (1959) also noted that olfactory hallucinations in some temporal lobe epileptic patients were followed by prolonged depressive episodes. Weil considered that the prolonged depression in such cases was due to the presence of a 'diffuse temporal lobe lesion'. Therefore, if the anterior lobectomy itself plays a significant part in the increased incidence of depression, one possible explanation may be that the subsequent gliosis and scar tissue formation in the temporal lobe remnant produces the so-called 'diffuse temporal lesion' implicated by Weil. Conversely, the rise in depression may only reflect the natural progression of the disease coinciding with the high rates of depression found at follow-up on *non-operated epileptics* (Henriksen, Juul-Jensen & Lund, 1970). Indeed, Taylor (1969a) remarked that the high suicide rate at five-year follow-up in severely handicapped epileptics simply attests to the seriousness of their interminable burden. Whatever its cause, however, the problem of post-operative depression would appear to be a significant feature in the long-term clinical management of lobectomy patients.

Incidence of aggression. Another significant feature in the clinical management of some temporal lobe epileptics is the problem of aggression, and although the violence of certain epileptics is notorious, epileptic aggression has attracted relatively few scientific studies (Trimble, 1981). In one report, Rey, Pond, and Evans (1949) found a pathological degree of irritability and aggression in 75 per cent of their patients, and Ounsted,

Table 12. *Incidence of depression: pre-operation and post-operation*

Diagnostic category	Pre-operation No. of cases	Post-operation No. of cases
Developmental lesion	0	1
Trauma	0	0
Alien tissue		
Astrocytic	0	0
Oligodendrocytic	0	0
Mixed glial	0	0
Neuronoglial		
(ganglioglial)	0	0
Neuronoglial		
(cortical dysplasia)	0	0
Vascular	0	1*
Ammon's horn sclerosis	0	7**
Inflammatory	0	0
Indefinite	0	2*
No apparent abnormality	1	9*
Double pathology	0	4*
Total	1 (0.4%)	24 (10%)
Total No. of cases pre-operation	247	
post-operation with F/U	234	

*denotes each patient who committed suicide
Percentage figures in brackets indicate incidence of depression

Lindsay, and Norman (1966) noted a high incidence of hyperactive and violent outbursts, especially in patients with early onset epilepsy who had suffered a cerebral insult. In addition, several authors have tried to correlate aggressive behaviour with abnormal limbic system activity, especially in relation to amygdala damage (Goddard, 1964; Mark & Ervin, 1970). However, Kligman and Goldberg (1975) reviewed the literature and severely criticized the design of many of the previous papers. They concluded: 'It is not at present possible to answer the question of whether there is an increased incidence of aggressive behaviour in temporal lobe epilepsy'.

The major problem of investigating violence in epilepsy is its measurement. In the present study patients were deemed excessively violent when the medical notes made regular reference to phrases such as 'extreme aggression' or 'very violent', on the assumption that episodes of unusual vitriol were more likely to be recorded than not. Nevertheless it may well be that some episodes of aggression were regarded as normal by a patient or his relatives and not mentioned. Similarly, aggressive behaviour may be seen in the automatisms of a temporal-lobe fit and its true nature misunderstood. Notwithstanding these difficulties, the clinical notes over a period of several years were usually consistent if excessive violence had been a problem, and in the follow-up review every patient acted as his own control so that a change in post-operative behaviour was not difficult to detect.

The incidence of aggression is detailed in Table 13. After operation the rate fell from 22 per cent to 16 per cent, which is a significant reduction at the level $P < 0.05$.

Any diminution in violence following lobectomy is welcome, yet the neuroanatomical pathways involved are uncertain. There is much evidence from animal experiments which implicates *bilateral* temporal ablation and, more particularly, bilateral removal of the amygdala in a reduction of aggression, but this is more marked in some species than in others and a few studies have reported increased savageness rather than placidity (Goddard, 1964). The position in human beings is at least as complex and has been detailed by Corsellis (1970b) in his review of the pathological anatomy of the temporal lobe and limbic areas. Corsellis noted that nearly all pathological processes and lesions fail to respect anatomical boundaries, and commented that it was therefore peculiarly difficult to assess the significance of an apparent link between clinical and pathological observations, particularly when both categories are complex and may be ill-defined. Nevertheless, the present study has confirmed the previous work by Taylor (1972), who found a *reduction* in aggression after unilateral lobectomy. There is no doubt that the temporal lobe is intimately involved in many aspects of human emotion, including aggression (Corsellis, 1970b, for detailed references), but whether or not there is a direct link between the operative removal of one temporal lobe and the subsequent observed reduction in aggression remains open to debate.

The incidence of schizophrenia. Another area of debate is the association between psychotic illness and epilepsy; this has been reviewed recently by Trimble (1981). He found that there were a number of situations in which psychotic experiences were associated with a fit. In many cases, however, these episodes were associated with EEG abnormalities and an altered

Table 13. *Incidence of aggression: pre-operation and post-operation*

Diagnostic category	Pre-operation No. of cases	Post-operation No. of cases
Developmental lesion	1	1
Trauma	2	2
Alien tissue		
Astrocytic	2	0
Oligodendrocytic	0	0
Mixed glial	2	0
Neuronoglial (ganglioglial)	0	1
Neuronoglial (cortical dysplasia)	4	3
Vascular	2	1
Ammon's horn sclerosis	32	16
Inflammatory	2	2
Indefinite	1	2
No apparent abnormality	6	7
Double pathology	2	2
Total No. of cases	56	37
Total No. of cases in sample	249	
Pre-operative incidence of aggression	56/249 (22%)	
Total No. of cases with F/U	234	
Post-operative incidence of aggression	37/234 (16%)	

level of consciousness. The idea that epilepsy may be related to a more prolonged form of psychosis has also been supported (Hill, 1953; Pond, 1957; Slater & Beard, 1963; Ounsted & Lindsay, 1981). Furthermore, studies of patients with temporal lobe epilepsy have suggested that the presence of a focal abnormality in the temporal lobe may predispose to the psychosis (Taylor, 1975; Jensen & Larsen, 1979).

The pre-operative and post-operative incidences of psychosis in patients from the present research are detailed in Table 14; they provide more information for the debate but shed little light on its outcome. Indeed, the information itself may be biased, first, because psychotic patients were not usually selected for operation particularly in the latter years of the study (Taylor, 1975), and secondly, because the use of psychiatric terminology in the clinical notes may not have been uniform. Nevertheless, before lobectomy sixteen patients were considered to be suffering from a schizophrenic illness and another three had an unspeci-

Table 14. *Incidence of schizophrenia: pre-operation and post-operation*

Diagnostic category	Pre-operation No. of cases	Post-operation No. of cases
Developmental lesion	1	0
Trauma	0	0
Alien tissue		
Astrocytic	1	0
Oligodendrocytic	0	0
Mixed glial	1	1
Neuronoglial (ganglioglial)	0	2
Neuronoglial (cortical dysplasia)	0	0
Vascular	1	0
Ammon's horn sclerosis	6	7
Inflammatory	0	0
Indefinite	1	1
No apparent abnormality	4	5
Double pathology	0	2
Total	15 (6%)	18 (7%)
Total No. of cases in sample	247	
Total No. of cases with post-operative F/U	234	

Percentage figures in brackets indicate incidence of schizophrenia

fied psychosis. Of the sixteen schizophrenic epileptics, eight were found at operation to have an Ammon's horn sclerosis, four had Indefinite or No apparent abnormality, three had an Alien tissue lesion and one had a Developmental lesion. These findings do not support the view that a focal temporal lobe abnormality specially predisposes to the development of an epileptic psychosis. After lobectomy the overall incidence of schizophrenia remained virtually unchanged, but the distribution of cases between the diagnostic groups altered, in that no less than four patients with a ganglioglial lesion became schizophrenic (Case Nos. 60, 99, 102, and 144). Case No. 60 and 144 had an Ammon's horn sclerosis as well as a ganglioglial lesion and were therefore classified in the Double pathology group. The figures are too small to draw conclusions but it is interesting to note that no other patients with Alien tissue lesions became psychotic after operation although three with a pre-operative psychosis and Alien tissue pathology lost their psychotic symptoms after lobectomy. In all, the interpretation of results is particularly difficult and the relationship, if any, between specific temporal lobe pathology and schizophrenia must await further study.

NEUROPATHOLOGICAL FEATURES

(a)   Classification and diagnosis

A modified system of neuropathological classification is the linchpin of the present investigation but the various clinico-pathological correlations which have been derived from its use are relevant only if the classification is valid and the individual histological diagnoses are correct.

Unfortunately, histological diagnosis is not an exact science; it is a visual interpretation of patterns based on the experience, training, and natural talent of the histopathologist. It is almost certainly measured best by some form of 'peer group' analysis undertaken informally between colleagues or more formally in 'diagnostic committees' such as the ones used for tumour diagnosis by the American National Academy of Sciences or by the WHO. Thus, when the coded histological slides had been examined by the author and compared with the original report it was comforting to find that the author's diagnosis differed from the original report in only two of the 249 cases (these are discussed later).

The original reports in the present series were compiled using terminology based on the two standard British text books, *Greenfield's Neuropathology* and Russell and Rubinstein's *Pathology of Tumours of the Nervous System*. In addition to these reference works, relevant original reports were also followed (Earle, Baldwin & Penfield, 1953; Falconer, Pond, Meyer & Woolf, 1953; Meyer, Falconer & Beck, 1954; Cavanagh, 1958; Margerison & Corsellis, 1966) in order to produce a reasonably standardized basis for diagnosis. Nevertheless, in the course of the present review the author became aware of certain ambiguities in the standard nomenclature such as those which gave an implied aetiology and prognosis to certain lesions not necessarily justified by the clinical outcome. Therefore the modified classification was designed to determine prognosis and aetiology more accurately. The new terminology affects, most particularly, the Group 3 (Alien tissue) lesions: indeed, the term 'Alien tissue lesion' was coined specifically to avoid such evocative terms as neoplasm, tumour, hamartoma, and so forth, which might be unhelpful or misleading. The main tenet of the classification is based on the principle that no diagnostic group is given a name which implies an aetiology unless the evidence for such aetiology is overwhelming. Thus Group 1 (Developmental lesions) includes only those abnormalities widely regarded as developmental. Similarly, Group 2 (Trauma) contains only those cases in which there was histological evidence of a cortical or white matter scar; a clinical history of head injury alone was not enough. Conversely, all those groups without a known aetiology have been described and labelled as accurately as possible, using terms which do not prejudge the eventual clinical behaviour. Patients with a scarred Ammon's horn have been termed Ammon's horn sclerotics (Group 4) in keeping with their classical name, and cases with more than one lesion have been classified simply as the Double pathology group (Group 8).

(b) Diagnostic difficulties

(i) Defects of tissue processing and staining

The earliest sections were prepared from celloidin-embedded material stained by the classical histopathological methods of Nissl, Mallory, Heidenhain Woelcke, Van Gieson, and so on, and were remarkably well preserved, considering that some were 25 years old. However, the mounting medium of many older slides had developed a yellowish discolouration which could present problems in diagnosis and in photography. Occasionally the mounting medium had dried out and a few specimens were so badly distorted that they had to be excluded from the series as there was no spare tissue available for reprocessing. In fact, the absence of spare fresh tissue from many of the cases precluded the use of the more modern techniques such as enzyme histochemistry, immunohistochemistry, and electron microscopy, which may have helped to diagnose the more difficult cases, especially those in the Alien tissue group (Bancroft & Stevens, 1982).

(ii) Problems of anatomy: site of the lesion

Another difficulty was the accurate mapping of the abnormal temporal lobe tissue which was seen most often in specimens from the early years of the study before standardized block taking procedures had been developed. In some of these cases the full extent of the lesion could not be assessed: others may have been diagnosed as 'No abnormality' even though a small localized abnormality might have been present in the tissue that had not been processed with one of the blocks of tissue prepared for histology. Nevertheless a reasonably accurate map of the site and extent of the lesion could be attempted for almost every patient.

The maps showed two significant correlations between neuropathological diagnosis and the location of the pathological abnormality. The first was that Alien tissue abnormalities occurred more often in the amygdaloid region ($P < 0.005$) and the second was the extremely common involvement of the amygdaloid region in the patients with sclerosis of the Ammon's horn ($P < 0.0001$).

(iii) Problems of anatomy: extent of surgical resection

Apart from the small number of patients with 'Indefinite pathology' it was not difficult to determine histologically whether the lesion had been removed completely at operation. Only 12 patients were considered to have had an incomplete resection of the lesion (Table 15). Interestingly, they fared significantly worse after operation than the remaining patients in the series in both the post-operative effect on fit frequency ($P < 0.1$) and also the post-operative effect on personality and social adjustment ($P < 0.01$). Moreover, no less than five of the twelve patients had died by the end of the survey and four of the deaths were attributed to a recurrence of the original pathology (see Table 9). The post-operative death rate was significantly higher in these patients at the level $P < 0.05$.

(iv) Errors of diagnosis

The cases which presented most difficulty were those with Indefinite pathology and a few patients with Alien tissue lesions. The problems in the Indefinite pathology group involved the definition of a precise borderline between the appearances of the normal temporal lobe and those lobes which were clearly abnormal. In practice, the diagnostic choice usually rested between 'no abnormality' and 'equivocal pathology', although there were a few cases where a clump of unusual cells, in the amygdaloid nucleus, suggested the diagnosis of an 'Alien tissue' lesion.

The diagnostic problems in patients with definite 'Alien tissue' pathology, however, concerned the accurate identification of specific cell types and it was in this category that the author produced one case in which the conclusion differed from that of the original report. This involved Case No. 153, originally reported as an 'Oligodendroglial abnormality with formations of hypertrophic *reactive* astrocytes reminiscent of clumps of blastomatous neuroglia that are frequently seen in the central form of

Table 15. *Results of surgery in patients with incomplete resection of temporal lobe lesion*

Diagnostic category	Case No.	Sex	Length of follow-up (yrs)	Effect of surgery on fits	Effect of surgery on personality and social adjustment	Comments
Astrocytic glial lesion	72	F	8	Worse	Unaltered	Died. Recurrence of lesion
	194	M	2	Worse	Unaltered	Died. Recurrence of lesion
	103	F	15	Worse	Unaltered	Died. Recurrence of lesion
Oligodendrocytic lesion	131	F	10	Worse	Unaltered	Developing a dense hemiparesis
	235	M	20	Worse	Unaltered	Died. Recurrence of lesion
	15	F	2	Fit-free	Normal life	
	48	M	17	Fit-free	Unaltered	Bizarre athetoid movements
Inflammatory lesion	130	M	3	Improved	Worse	Died in a fit
	193	F	12	Unaltered	Unaltered	
	214	F	6	Improved	Improved	
	247	M	5	Unaltered	Unaltered	Dysphasic. In institutional care
	249	F	No f/u	—	—	

von Recklinghausen's neurofibromatosis (Cavanagh, 1958, Case No. 5). The present author felt that the lesion consisted of a complex mixture of abnormal oligodendroglial and abnormal astrocytic cells and therefore classed the lesion as a Mixed glial abnormality; a discrepancy merely involving the interpretation of the astrocytic element of the lesion. The other diagnostic difference concerned Case No. 91, which had been reported originally as 'No abnormality'. However, at the medial edge of the resected specimen there was a small mass of abnormal glia consisting of a mixture of astrocytes and oligodendroglial cells. This case was therefore also diagnosed as a Mixed glial abnormality. In the remaining 247 cases, the author's view agreed with the original.

(c) Diagnostic groups

Group 1. Developmental abnormalities

The act of birth marks no particular milestone in the development of the human brain and many years must elapse before structural maturity is achieved (Norman, 1963). Thus, in the widest sense, developmental disorders include all those instances where the process of normal brain development is disturbed, whether early in prenatal life or later on in childhood. However, the developing nervous system does not always respond to injury in the same way as mature tissue, and it is therefore difficult to determine the exact aetiology of many malformations, particularly when animal experiments have shown that the same lesion may be produced both by genetic and environmental causes (Norman, 1963) and when early interference with development is known to produce a much more catastrophic response than later injury (Wertham & Wertham, 1934). For this reason it has been customary to classify developmental abnormalities by their structural features without implicating aetiology, and the present author has followed the same procedure.

Urich (1976) reviewed the developmental malformations and noted their complexity, and the value of animal experiments in understanding some aspects of pathogenesis (Hicks, 1952; Kalter, 1968, Elizan & Fabiyi, 1970). However he concluded that the cause of many developmental malformations in man is largely undetermined.

The role of developmental abnormalities in the causation of temporal lobe epilepsy is equally uncertain. Jensen and Klinken (1976) have summarized the published histological data from temporal lobectomy patients along with the results of their Danish series. Most histological studies have not been elaborate; indeed, apart from the Danish material, the only detailed neuropathology with long-term clinical follow-up has been published by the Guy's, Maudsley group on patients who form part of the present series (Meyer, Falconer & Beck, 1954; Cavanagh, 1958;

Falconer, Serafetinides & Corsellis, 1964; Corsellis, 1970a). Even the Danish study of 74 cases is not comprehensively illustrated and they do not have a specific group for 'Developmental' lesions. Nevertheless, among their illustrated cases there are at least four examples of typical developmental anomalies (a minimum incidence of 6.4 per cent). In the present series, however. Developmental abnormalities formed the smallest group, only 2.4 per cent of the sample. There were six patients, four with cystic lesions and two with cortical malformations. One patient (Case No. 57) had an Ammon's horn sclerosis as well as a cystic lesion and was included in the Double pathology group. The cystic lesions were of various types; an arachnoid cyst, an epidermoid cyst and two simple cysts situated in the white matter anterior to, but separate from, the inferior horn of the ventricle. The last two lesions were surrounded by a relatively thick layer of neuroglial tissue and one had an inner lining of ependyma. The two cortical abnormalities showed small areas of polymicrogyric cortex distorting the inferior temporal gyrus. One of these (Case No. 59) also had nodules of heterotopic grey matter in the white matter ventral to the inferior horn.

From this account it may be seen that the pathology of the developmental lesions is very diverse; their causation is probably similar. No patient had a recorded history of birth injury and only one had a recorded head injury (Case No. 59). Another patient had febrile convulsions and a subsequent bout of status epilepticus; his temporal lobe showed an Ammon's horn sclerosis as well as a white-matter cyst. The group as a whole were the last to develop fits (mean age 22 years, $P < 0.01$) a surprising fact explained possibly by the small number or perhaps by the relative indolence of the lesions. They were unaffected by operation, despite the fact that all six abnormalities were thought to have been removed completely by the surgery. However, developmental lesions in the brain and elsewhere may be multiple, and it is impossible to be certain that a resection of one temporal lobe had removed every lesion.

It may be contended that the rarity of the developmental abnormalities and their unresponsiveness to treatment suggests that they are 'incidental' to the patient's epilepsy. Indeed this contention is impossible to refute for although major neural abnormalities account for only 0.6 per cent of the total births (Carter, David & Laurence, 1968) the total incidence of neural malformations may be considerably higher (Crome & Stern, 1972). However it is also equally possible that an 'incidental' lesion may become, later, an epileptogenic focus. Thus the presence of a temporal lobe lesion, whatever its cause, may be argued as circumstantial evidence of its involvement with the epileptic process.

In summary, therefore, developmental abnormalities are a rare and diverse collection in temporal lobectomy material. They give rise to epilepsy which starts, most often, in early adult life and their removal does not appear to alter significantly the natural course of the patient's epileptic illness.

Group 2. Trauma

An association between head injury, brain damage, and epilepsy has been known for centuries. However, the complex changes which may result from such head injuries have only more recently begun to be understood (Jakob, 1914; Holbourn, 1943; Pudenz & Sheldon, 1946; Unterharnscheidt & Higgins, 1969; Lindenberg, 1971; Strich, 1976; Hume Adams, 1984), and it is clear from these reports that brain damage may occur in a number of ways. First, the brain may be bruised and lacerated at the site of impact; secondly, the brain may rotate within the skull, tearing nerve fibres and producing contre-coup injury at sites away from the initial blow; and thirdly, a decrease in intracranial pressure may cause cavitation of cerebral tissue with release of gas bubbles. Furthermore, the brain may be damaged by secondary systemic factors such as hypoxia, brain swelling, hypotension, and fat embolism which may all accompany the initial trauma.

The temporal lobe may be involved in all these varieties of injury and the detailed mechanisms of contusion, laceration, and contre-coup damage as they affect the lobe have been drawn explicitly by Courville (1957). He studied acute lesions and found that they were most common after 'closed' injuries sustained with the head in motion and were usually located on the lateral surface, the orbital surface, or at the temporal pole; they rarely affected the uncus or parahippocampal gyrus. Courville also reviewed 113 cases of old temporal-lobe trauma verified at post-mortem. Epileptic fits had been recorded in 21 per cent (33 cases) but grand mal fits were most common (18 cases); whereas combined grand mal and psychomotor fits occurred in 11 cases; 'pure' psychomotor fits occurred in only three patients. He concluded that although temporal lobe contusions were common, 'pure' psychomotor seizures rarely complicated the lesion.

In the present study, 10 of the 249 patients (4 per cent of the total sample) showed histological evidence of cerebral trauma and eight of these suffered grand mal fits as well as frequent psychomotor attacks. These eight cases had 'blunt' injuries, mostly without skull fracture, although many were regarded clinically as 'severe'. The remaining two patients (Case Nos. 22 and 209) exhibited 'pure' psychomotor fits and interestingly these two patients were the only two with a true 'penetrating' injury, one by the blades from a pair of scissors and the second by a fragment of shrapnel. The findings support Roberts's (1979) general statement that head injuries complicated by brain penetration are more likely to give rise to focal attacks, whereas uncomplicated injuries give rise to a higher proportion of generalized convulsions.

Eight of the ten 'Trauma group' patients had a corroborating clinical history of head injury ($P < 0.0001$) which contrasts sharply with the findings of Jensen and Klinken (1976) who found no correlation between their neuropathological findings and head injury. However, this may be explained by their choice of histological groups, which divided cases into: (1) Focal lesions including small tumours and well-defined non-neoplastic changes; (2) Gliosis (nodular and diffuse); (3) Perivascular infiltration; (4) Equivocal changes; and (5) Iatrogenic insult. These are not specific neuropathological entities and may have resulted in overlap of one diagnostic group with another, thus masking any positive statistical correlation.

Nine of the ten patients in the present series showed focal scar formation with a variable degree of cortical nerve cell loss and fibrous gliosis. The surrounding temporal lobe white matter was always gliosed, sometimes intensely, often with considerable demyelination. The remaining patient (Case No. 2) had a subdural hygroma removed at lobectomy and the histological appearances were those of thickened and congested leptomeninges overlying the temporal convexity. Three patients had Double pathology, the second lesion in each case being an Ammon's horn sclerosis.

The distribution of the focal scarring varied but the middle and inferior temporal gyri were the areas most commonly affected.

The clinical and neuropathological findings show a high correlation between the histological evidence of cerebral trauma and a clinical history of head injury. It is also clear that in addition to the focal cortical damage, these patients always show widespread white matter damage spreading almost certainly beyond the confines of the resected lobe. It is therefore not surprising that the long-term effects of lobectomy were not good. The results show that the operation does not affect statistically the fit pattern, whereas their psychiatric and social adjustment to life is statistically worse ($P < 0.05$). It therefore appears, both from an empirical examination of the results, and from a neuropathological examination of the brain, that patients with severe post-traumatic epilepsy are best excluded from lobectomy surgery.

Group 3. Alien tissue lesions

The difficulties of defining a 'tumour' or 'neoplasm' are not confined to lesions within the central nervous system; indeed, they have concerned general pathologists for nearly a century. Nicholson (1925) was brave enough to consider the definition impossible. 'Wherever we look we see that tumours exhibit no differences in kind, but only differences in degree

– and these often the slightest – from the tissues in the body. I have tried for years to formulate a definition but have failed.' Willis (1947) ventured what he considered was a satisfactory definition: 'A tumour is an abnormal mass of tissue, the growth of which exceeds and is uncoordinated with that of normal tissues, and persists in the same excessive manner after cessation of the stimuli which evoked the change'.

However, over 30 years later the World Health Organization Committee on Central Nervous System Tumours was still struggling with terminology (World Health Organization, 1979). Russell and Rubinstein (1977) aptly summarized the current position in the introduction to their book: 'A somewhat arbitrary line must be drawn between what should be included or excluded under the title *Tumours of the Nervous System*. Debatable points arise both topographically and in the interpretation of the word tumour'. They go on to say 'within our conception of neoplastic disease we have found it necessary to give considerable attention to a variety of lesions that are of a maldevelopmental character, conveniently termed hamartoma. Some of these are virtually inseparable from the true neoplasms, both in their structure and behaviour'.

Every study of temporal lobectomy has included a number of patients with small focal lesions which invite the histological label of 'neoplasm' yet their very presence in patients selected for lobectomy suggests that they have been causing fits for years, if not decades, without obvious increase in size or disturbance of the surrounding tissues. In addition, clinical experience has shown that many of these lesions may be removed completely without signs of recurrence. On the other hand, some of their number behave like typical neoplasms with recurrence and eventual death of the patient concerned.

These small focal lesions have been described over the years (Falconer, Pond, Meyer & Woolf, 1953; Cavanagh, 1958; Edgar and Baldwin, 1960; Falconer, Serafetinides & Corsellis, 1964; Jann Brown, 1973; Jensen & Klinken, 1976), and vary from a small cluster of rather indolent cells to a bizarre aggregation of cells which appear wildly 'neoplastic'. Cavanagh (1958) began his thoughtful paper by suggesting that the lesions represented pathological changes at an earlier stage of development than might normally be expected at post-mortem, implying the possibility that they represented the first stages of a neoplasm, but he concluded that they behaved as hamartomas which might be considered as possible potential points for the further development of gliomas. However, Cavanagh was only able to study eight cases, too few to consider the suggestion that some varieties were hamartomatous whilst others might be neoplastic. Jann Brown (1973) and Jensen and Klinken (1976) also studied the small focal lesions, but followed, essentially, the conclusions of Cavanagh.

Forty-nine focal abnormalities were present in the current study (including 11 with Double pathology), which represents some 20 per cent of the total sample. Jann Brown (1973) found an incidence of 18 per cent whilst Jensen and Klinken observed an incidence of 5.4 per cent. On initial examination the lesions were labelled according to traditional nomenclature using such terms as astrocytoma, mixed glial tumour, ganglioglioma, haemangioma calcificans, but following the delineation of another specific group of curious neuronoglial lesions termed 'cortical dysplasia' (Taylor, Falconer, Bruton & Corsellis, 1971), the present author considered that there was such confusion that the classical terms were unhelpful. Therefore all lesions in the present group were described purely by cell type without prejudging their eventual behaviour. They then easily fell into three categories; glial lesions, neuronoglial lesions and vascular abnormalities, according to the tissue element involved. A generic name for the whole group was considered and the term 'Alien tissue lesion' was chosen, using 'Alien' in the sense of foreign or strange. In every case, particular attention was paid to variations in histological appearance, such as cellular pleomorphism, presence of mitoses, and calcification of tissue, to try to determine whether these affected the prognosis after surgery.

In the following section each of the Alien tissue subgroups will be discussed separately, after which the results of the histological analysis will be presented briefly.

Group 3(a). Glial lesions

I. Astrocytic glial lesions. Astrocytes were recognized originally by Virchow (1846), but their detailed investigation awaited the development of selective stains (Ramón y Cajal, 1913, 1916; del Rio Hortega, 1919, 1921); modifications of these metallic impregnation stains still form an important part of the assessment of glial abnormalities. Nevertheless the emphasis of glial cell investigation has turned more recently to the newer techniques of electron microscopy, immunocytochemistry and tissue culture, involving both normal astrocytic structure and its reaction to disease (Peters & Palay, 1965; Palay, 1966; Nathaniel & Nathaniel, 1981; Eng & DeArmond, 1982).

Astrocytes may also be involved in neoplastic change, and astrocytic tumours form approximately 20 per cent of gliomas (Russell & Rubinstein, 1977). These authors recognized protoplasmic, fibrillary, pilocytic, gemistocytic, and anaplastic varieties of atrocytoma and discussed their association with the much more commonly occurring glioblastoma multiforme. In the context of histological diagnosis Russell and Rubinstein (1977) reviewed also the characteristics of 'anaplasia' and 'tumour grading' (Kernohan, Mabon, Svien & Adson, 1949). They considered that the principle of tumour grading, if used at all, should be restricted to autopsy material when the whole tumour could be sampled. The problem of tumour grading has been echoed more recently by the World Health Organization Committee on C.N.S. tumours (WHO, 1979).

With this in mind, the assessment of astrocytic lesions in the present material has not been burdened by the necessity to predict malignancy or even neoplasia by eye alone. The important feature is an accurate identification of each cell type with a comment on the extent of other features which include cellular pleomorphism, abnormal vascular proliferation, mitotic rate, tissue necrosis, and calcification.

Nine patients had a temporal lobe abnormality composed entirely of astrocytic glia which represented 3.6 per cent of the total sample and 18.3 per cent of the Alien tissue lesions. In eight cases the lesion was identifiable as a discrete mass; the remaining patient (Case No. 194) had a diffuse infiltration of abnormal glia throughout the lobe. One specimen (Case No. 147) had Double pathology, the second lesion being an Ammon's horn sclerosis. The distribution of the abnormalities varied within the lobe; most lesions were found in the parahippocampal gyrus and the amygdaloid region.

The histological appearances also varied from case to case; in Case No. 42 the abnormality consisted almost entirely of mature protoplasmic astrocytes arranged in a loose cystic network, whilst the predominant cell of Case No. 17 was a spindle-shaped, hyperchromatic fibrillary astrocyte. Other cases were more pleomorphic, especially Case No. 147, in which there were numerous, bizarre, giant astrocytes, many of them multinucleated. Five cases showed some degree of abnormal vascular proliferation within the astrocytic lesion, although there was no tissue necrosis, pseudopalisading, or calcification. In addition, there were no mitoses, and no statistical association was found between any of these histological features and the outcome after lobectomy.

All but two of the abnormalities were considered, histologically, to have been removed at operation. These two patients (Case Nos. 72 and 194) died from a recurrence of the lesion some eight years and two years respectively after lobectomy. At the end of the survey, all the remaining seven patients were still alive, the average length of follow-up being seven years.

Clinically, the astrocytic glial lesions gave rise to late-onset epilepsy (mean age at first fit 27.25 years), which, even compared with other Alien tissue subgroups, is highly significant at the level of $P < 0.002$. In the group as a whole, the post-operative data show no statistical change in fit pattern or psychosocial adjustment after lobectomy.

Within the group, the combination of late-onset epilepsy and the recurrence of certain lesions suggest that they are acquired and behave as neoplasms rather than as hamartomatous maldevelopments. However, the fact that seven of the original nine cases were still alive after an average of seven years suggests that the behaviour of the lesions is very benign.

II. Oligodendrocytic glial lesions. Oligodendroglial cells were identified first by Robertson (1899) and formed one part of Ramón y Cajal's 'third element' of the neuroglia (Ramón y Cajal, 1909). They were described further and named by del Rio Hortega (1921) because of their appearance in metallic impregnation stains. Oligodendrocytes are the commonest glial component of the nervous system, arranged usually as satellite cells to the neurons, or in rows between the neural fibres (Peters, Palay & Webster, 1976). As their name implies they have few branching processes, and a round or oval nucleus. They react commonly by undergoing 'acute swelling' with vacuolation, expansion of the cytoplasm, and pyknosis of the nucleus. The final picture is that of an enlarged, rounded cell, with a well-marked cytoplasmic membrane, more or less 'empty' cytoplasm, and a nucleus which appears to float. Like astrocytes, the oligodendroglia undergo neoplastic change and the 'acute swelling' gives a characteristic appearance to the tumour (Russell & Rubinstein, 1977). The tumour cells are arranged frequently as compact masses of these empty swollen cells intersected by a scanty stroma of blood vessels and connective tissue. Mucinous degeneration of the tumour cells may occur with mucin-filled microcysts being another common feature. The final component of many lesions is calcification, with calcium salts deposited in the walls of the intrinsic blood vessels.

The first oligodendroglial tumours were recognized by Bailey and Bucy (1929). They are found in the cerebral hemispheres in adult life, with a peak age incidence of 40 years (Zülch, 1956). In general they are relatively uncommon compared with astrocytic lesions and form approximately 5 per cent of gliomas (Russell & Rubinstein, 1977).

In the present study six patients had oligodendroglial lesions. The patients represent only 2.4 per cent of the total sample but 12 per cent of the Alien tissue lesions. One patient (Case No. 131) had an Ammon's horn sclerosis and was assigned also to the Double pathology group. All but one abnormality (Case No. 58) was visible on initial examination of the lobe, and more commonly in the medial and dorso-medial part. All six lesions involved the amygdaloid nucleus, while the uncus and superior temporal gyrus were also affected in three cases. In contrast, the middle and inferior temporal gyri were spared and the fusiform and parahippo-campal gyrus were involved only once. Histology, however, showed that most cases spread more widely within the temporal lobe white matter, the exception being Case No. 58. The oligodendroglial cells which made up the abnormality were usually well differentiated with oval nuclei and clear cytoplasm separated by a delicate connective tissue stroma. There were no visible mitoses, no tissue necrosis, and no abnormal vascular proliferation, and only one case (Case No. 131) showed any degree of cellular pleomorphism. Similarly only one case (Case No. 103) was calcified but microcystic degeneration was much more common and involved four of the six cases (Case Nos. 103, 160, 216, and 235).

The more important feature, however, was that only three of the lesions were considered, histologically, to have been removed completely at operation. In the remaining three cases (Case Nos. 103, 131, and 235) abnormal oligodendroglial cells were visible at the extreme dorso-medial edge of the resected specimen. Case Nos. 103 and 235 died from a recurrence of the lesion some 15 and 20 years respectively after operation. The latest available information on Case No. 131 (10 years after lobectomy) is that her fits have recurred and that she has recently developed a left hemiparesis.

Clinically, the oligodendroglial lesions give rise to late onset epilepsy (mean age at first fit 26 years) which, when compared with other Alien tissue subgroups, is significant at the level $P < 0.01$. The post-operative data show no significant statistical difference in fit pattern or psychosocial adjustment after lobectomy. However, two patients eventually died from a recurrence of the lesion.

Thus, in common with the pure astrocytic lesions, the oligodendroglial abnormalities combine the features of late-onset epilepsy and recurrence of the lesion if not completely resected. They therefore behave as neoplasms, but appear to be even more slowly progressive than their astrocytic counterparts.

III. Mixed glial abnormalities.   The third variety of glial abnormality in the current series has been a diagnostic dilemma for many years (Rubinstein, 1972; Russell & Rubinstein, 1977). Indeed, in the Introduction to the *American Armed Forces Atlas of Tumour Pathology*, Rubinstein (1972) states that 'the presence of mixed tumour cell populations often presents difficulties that may defy attempts at classification and prognosis'. He describes three types of lesion; 'In one group of tumours it involves solely the gliogenous elements: these are the mixed gliomas. In the second group, both neuronal and glial cell forms appear to participate in the neoplastic process: these are the gangliogliomas. In the third group both gliomatous and sarcomatous cells are found in contiguity or closely intermingled: these are the mixed gliomas and sarcomas'.

Rubinstein appears to favour the view that the 'Mixed Gliomas' have an oligodendroglial origin with abnormal astrocytic elements contained within the lesion. He states that 'Oligodendrogliomas often contain glial elements that are recognisably not oligodendroglial. These may include fibrillary or protoplasmic astrocytes, gemistocytes, astroblasts or spongioblasts ... Basically, however, their behaviour is usually that of an oligodendroglioma. ... Aside from the close intermingling of the various cell forms, oligodendrogliomas not infrequently contain distinct foci of pure astrocytoma'.

The 'mixed glial abnormalities' described in the present temporal lobe material correspond histologically to the 'mixed gliomas' described above, in that they are composed of a mixture of abnormal astrocytes and abnormal oligodendroglial cells within the same lesion. Their 13 members form 5.2 per cent of the series and are the largest subgroup of the Alien tissue lesions (26.5 per cent). Only one lobe (Case No. 91) was considered normal on naked-eye examination, and histologically the lesions involved, most often, the amygdaloid region (7 cases). Every lesion was composed of a mixture of abnormal oligodendroglial and abnormal astrocytic cells, but within this basic framework there was a considerable difference of structural emphasis. The cellular pleomorphism and nuclear hyperchromasia varied from case to case but there were no mitoses. Unlike the monoglial lesions the great majority of cases were calcified and some specimens contained large numbers of calcospherites (Case Nos. 69, 104, 133, 181 and 208). Similarly, the presence of microcystic spaces varied from patient to patient; two lobes (Case Nos. 137 and 164) contained large cystic lesions within which the glial abnormality appeared to arise. These cystic lesions were lined by a single layer of plump glia and had the appearances of a simple developmental cyst. These two cases, along with two others which showed a sclerotic Ammon's horn (Case Nos. 207 and 240) were classified also in the Double pathology group.

Another variable feature of the mixed glial group was the amount of vascular tissue in the connective tissue stroma separating the glial cells. In three cases (Case Nos. 69, 153 and 181) this vascular proliferation was so plentiful that the cases were typical of those described originally as 'Haemangioma Calcificans' by Penfield and Ward (1948).

The lesions of all 13 patients were thought to have been removed completely at operation and only one patient (Case No. 91) has died since lobectomy, from a cause unrelated to his operation; in no case has there been a recurrence of the primary mass.

Clinically, the mixed glial lesions give rise to epilepsy, which begins at a young age (mean age at first fit 10.58 years). The average length of follow-up since lobectomy is 13 years and 11 of the 13 patients are fit and well at the time of this study. The post-operative results show a significant improvement in fit frequency for the group as a whole at the level $P < 0.005$. However, the personality and social adjustment after operation is not significantly changed.

Thus it may be seen that the mixed glial lesions differ markedly from their pure astrocytic and pure oligodendroglial counterparts. First, the epilepsy begins at a much younger age; secondly, the lesion is often heavily calcified and on two occasions appears to arise in association with a large developmental cyst. Thirdly, there is no evidence of recurrence of the primary pathology, and finally, the operation results in a significant reduction in the frequency of epileptic fits.

Combining these features together it is tempting to suggest that the mixed glial lesions in the temporal lobe are developmental in origin rather than neoplastic.

Group 3(b).   Neuronoglial lesions

This group of Alien tissue lesions includes all patients whose temporal lobe abnormality contains abnormal nerve cells and abnormal glia in the same lesion. The diagnosis was never confirmed unless the abnormal nerve cell element showed unmistakable Nissl substance and neurofibrils demonstrable by an appropriate silver impregnation. A total of 17 patients (6.8 per cent of the sample) had abnormalities of this type but from a cursory examination of the lesions it became evident that two quite distinct varieties of neuropathology were involved. The first type (nine cases) corresponded well with the well-recognized entity of 'ganglioglioma' first described by Courville (1930). The second (eight cases) typified the abnormality described as 'Cortical Dysplasia' by Taylor, Falconer, Bruton, and Corsellis (1971).

The putative origin and distribution of the 'gangliogliomas' was discussed in detail by Rubinstein (1972). He considered the possibility that they were hamartomatous, but thought it more likely that they were slow-growing tumours in which, rarely, anaplastic transformation occurred in the glial element. They were situated in the region of the third ventricle and the hypothalamus, or in the temporal lobe where they could produce longstanding epilepsy.

The second category of neuronoglial abnormalities clearly differed neuropathologically from the gangliogliomas and formed a part of the series of ten cases termed 'Cortical Dysplasia' reported by Taylor, Falconer, Bruton and Corsellis in 1971. In their original series there were five temporal lobectomy specimens, ablations from three frontal lobes, from one occipital and from one parietal lobe. The lesions were often invisible to naked-eye examination but the histology was similar in each case. This consisted of clusters of bizarre, giant neurons littered through all but the first cortical layer. In addition, there were grotesque cells, probably of glial origin, in the molecular layer and the depths of the affected cortex as well as in the subjacent white matter. The abnormality was thought to be a malformation and the authors distinguished it on clinical and pathological grounds from other defined conditions and in particular from tuberous sclerosis. Both groups of neuronoglial lesions will now be considered separately.

(i) 'Ganglioglial lesions'.   There were nine patients in the group (3.6 per cent of the sample), four with Double pathology (Case Nos. 10, 60, 98, and 144). Their histological features resembled that of the mixed glial abnormalities, the only additional feature being the presence of abnormal and often giant nerve cells, resembling ganglion cells, scattered within the lesion. These aberrant nerve cells contained Nissl substance and neuro-

fibrils; they occurred in variable numbers mixed with the clusters of abnormal astrocytes and oligodendroglia. Most lesions were calcified (Case Nos. 7, 10, 102, 144, 162 and 230); three patients had an additional Ammon's horn sclerosis (Case Nos. 10, 60, and 144), and one abnormality occurred in the presence of a large ependymal-lined cyst (Case No. 98). Every lesion showed some degree of cellular pleomorphism and this was moderately severe in Case Nos. 98 and 99. In addition, four cases had abnormal proliferation in the connective tissue stroma separating the glial clusters (Case Nos. 99, 144, 162, and 230). However, there was no tissue necrosis and no mitotic activity. Most of the abnormalities were situated in the uncus, amygdaloid nucleus, hippocampus, or parahippocampal gyrus. In only one patient (Case No. 98) were the lateral temporal gyri involved. All lesions were thought to have been removed completely at operation and after an average of nine years no patient has shown any evidence of a recurrence.

Clinically, the ganglioglial lesions give rise to early-onset epilepsy (mean age 6.44 years) with no obvious precipitating cause, and all patients were judged psychologically normal prior to lobectomy. However, the post-operative results in the group differed in certain respects from any other. There was a significant reduction in fit frequency ($P < 0.05$) resembling that of the mixed glial category, but the personality and social adjustment in the group as a whole was not significantly altered. In particular, of the six patients whose personality and social adjustment were worse after lobectomy, no less than four became schizophrenic (Case Nos. 60, 99, 102, and 144) and the other two (Case Nos. 10 and 230) were aggressive and unmanageable. One of the schizophrenics committed suicide (Case No. 144) and another (Case No. 102) is in permanent psychiatric care. The occurrence of post-operative psychiatric illness is not statistically significant, possibly because of the small numbers of the group, but such a tendency is not seen elsewhere. In this respect the ganglioglial group results differ from the closely allied mixed glial category.

In summary, therefore, it would appear that the ganglioglial lesions, in the temporal lobe at least, behave clinically as developmental lesions rather than true neoplasms. They give rise to fits in early childhood, and show no evidence of recurrence many years after lobectomy. In addition, one case occurred in association with a large 'developmental' cyst and three others occurred in conjunction with an Ammon's horn sclerosis. In these latter three cases it is tempting to suggest that the ganglioglial lesion initiated the epileptic seizures, with the subsequent development of hippocampal sclerosis.

In all these features, as well as the significant post-operative reduction in fit frequency, the ganglioglial lesions behave like the mixed glial abnormalities. The main difference is the rather surprising, but not

statistically significant, finding concerning the post-operative development of a schizophrenic illness or a severe behavioural disorder in six of
the nine patients in the group. This finding is not paralleled in the mixed
glial group, and in neuropathological terms the only differences between
the groups are the presence of the abnormal 'ganglion-like' nerve cells
and the tendency of the ganglioglial lesions to occur more frequently in
the amygdaloid and hippocampal region. The explanation for the differences is unclear and it must be stressed again that the ganglioglial group
comprised only nine cases. Nevertheless, it would seem that the results
would provide interesting material for future research.

(ii)   Cortical dysplasia.   The second type of neuronoglial abnormality
occurred in eight patients (3.2 per cent of the sample) and by definition
their histological lesion was also composed of a mixture of abnormal
nerve cells and abnormal glia. However, in other respects the neuropathological features differed greatly from the ganglioglial abnormalities. Six
of the eight specimens (Case Nos. 141, 174, 182, 213, 217, and 238)
showed no naked-eye abnormality and in the two remaining patients
(Case Nos. 65 and 66) the lesion was visible only as a blurring of the
normally sharp demarcation between the grey and white matter of the
affected area. In addition no case showed Double pathology.

Microscopically, the abnormality was identified by a disturbance in the
normal cortical architecture produced by the presence of a variable
number of huge, abnormally stained nerve cells which impregnated
deeply with silver. These cells had large nuclei, often with crescentic
thickening of the nuclear membrane and large quantities of deeply
staining Nissl substance. The deeper cortical layers and adjacent white
matter contained in addition other large abnormal cells with huge
hyperchromatic nuclei and frosted-glass-like cytoplasm, which most
closely resembled huge aberrant astrocytes. In addition, a few inter-
mediate cell forms between the abnormal neurons and abnormal glia were
seen. There was no evidence of calcification, microcyst formation, or
abnormal vascular proliferation and, despite the bizarre cellular pleomorphism, there were no mitoses. The abnormality involved the superior
temporal gyrus most often, with the middle and inferior temporal gyri
also commonly affected. In contrast, the uncus was completely spared,
and the amygdaloid nucleus, hippocampus, and parahippocampal gyrus
were involved only once each. All lesions were thought to have been
removed completely by the lobectomy and there has been no evidence of
recurrence after an average follow-up of eight years. The histological
appearances in all eight patients were typical of those described as focal
dysplasia of the cerebral cortex (Taylor, Falconer, Bruton & Corsellis,
1971). Indeed four cases in the present series (Case Nos. 65, 141, 213, and
217) were part of the 1971 paper. The remaining lesions were identified in
subsequent lobectomy patients.

Clinically the focal dysplasias give rise to epilepsy beginning in early adult life (mean age at first fit 14.75 years) which is significantly later than the ganglioglial lesions ($P < 0.05$). Post-operatively there was no significant alteration in fit pattern, unlike the ganglioglial lesions. The post-operative personality and social adjustment was also not significantly altered, with no tendency to develop psychiatric illness.

In certain respects, therefore, the focal cortical dysplasias differ from the ganglioglial lesions. They both behave as developmental lesions yet show a statistically significant discrepancy in respect of age at first fit. Indeed a similar discrepancy is seen between these lesions and the Group 1 (Developmental abnormality) patients in which the average age at first fit is even older (22.8 years). Furthermore, the response to lobectomy is different in that the ganglioglial lesions show definite improvement in post-operative fit frequency, whereas the focal dysplasias as a group and the Group 1 Developmental abnormalities do not. Notwithstanding these differences, however, the behaviour of the cortical dysplasias is that of a developmental anomaly in which a population of abnormal neurons and abnormal glia underlies the development of the temporal lobe fits.

Group 3(c). Vascular abnormalities

This is the smallest section of the Alien tissue lesions and is represented by four patients (1.6 per cent of the series). One patient (Case No. 28) also had a sclerotic Ammon's horn and was classified in the Double pathology category.

The common histological feature in each case was the presence, in the temporal cortex or white matter, of a mass of abnormal vascular tissue which resembled one of the well documented cerebral 'angiomatous malformations' (Russell & Rubinstein, 1977). Three of the four patients (Case Nos. 30, 32, and 188) were classical examples of a 'cavernous angioma' with a honeycomb of variably sized, thin-walled spaces filled with blood and separated from one another by thin fibrous strands. Some areas were thrombosed and there were even a few areas of calcification. The surrounding brain tissue was moderately gliosed and contained numbers of haemosiderin-laden macrophages suggesting old haemorrhage.

The fourth lesion (Case No. 28) was different, in that it was contained in an area of thickened leptomeninges overlying the middle temporal gyrus and was composed of a network of abnormally thickened arteries and veins. The calibre and thickness of these vessels varied greatly and the wall of one artery was so thick that it resembled a leiomyomatous nodule. The lesion was surrounded by numerous free-lying red cells suggesting recent haemorrhage. The appearances were those of a typical arterio-venous malformation.

In no lesion, however, was there any sign of cellular pleomorphism and there were no visible mitoses.

A study of the vascular malformations in patients with temporal lobe epilepsy was made by Edgar and Baldwin in 1960. Their paper illustrates clearly the problem of nomenclature in temporal lobe pathology. They found ten 'arterio-venous' malformations representing an incidence of 11.4 per cent in a series of 88 temporal lobectomies. They subdivided the abnormalities by anatomical site rather than histological appearance to produce an 'intracerebral' and a 'meningocortical' group. Histology of the lesions, however, shows a mixture of cavernous haemangiomas and arterio-venous malformation. They then compared the 'intracerebral' lesions with 'Haemangioma calcificans' and the 'meningocortical' lesions with the 'cryptic hamartomas', thus attempting a comparison between an anatomical site on the one hand and a histological entity on the other. In contrast, Russell and Rubinstein (1977) chose histological appearances as the basis of classification. They discussed the differences between the 'true neoplasms' of blood vessels and the 'angiomatous malformations' and stated that while the malformations were not truly neoplastic, it was clear that some grow and inflict progressive destruction on the surrounding brain. They believed that the evolution of vascular hamartomas occurs by progressive dilatation of blood vessels, leading to stenosis and thrombosis which may inflict further parenchymal damage on the adjacent cortex. In this context it is of note that all four abnormalities in the present series show histological evidence which suggests a recent or old bleed at the periphery of the lesion.

Clinically, the small number of patients with vascular lesions makes generalization difficult. However, on average the age at first fit was 14.5 years, and there were no obvious predisposing factors. All lesions were visible at operation and all were thought to have been removed completely after lobectomy. Statistically, there was no apparent post-operative alteration in fit pattern or social adjustment and no evidence of a recurrence after an average follow-up period of five years. Post-operatively one of the four patients became dysphasic, deteriorated intellectually, and was unable to work. Another (Case No. 32) became depressed and committed suicide two years after the operation.

In conclusion, the vascular lesions are difficult to summarize; they resemble malformations and do not appear to recur. However, they all show some suggestion of previous bleeding, which gives support to the belief (Russell & Rubinstein, 1977) that they tend to 'evolve' rather than to remain inert.

Histological features of the Alien tissue subgroups and their effect on long-term prognosis.   Histological material from the 49 members of the Alien tissue group was studied to compare variations in cellular morphology with the long-term outcome after surgery.

In this respect, six cellular features were examined:

(i)   Cellular pleomorphism
(ii) Presence of mitoses

(iii) Calcification of tissue
(iv) Abnormal vascular proliferation
(v) Tissue necrosis
(vi) Cyst formation.

(i) Cellular pleomorphism. This was assessed as absent, slight, moderate, or severe. Where no cellular pleomorphism was present, the glial, nerve cell, and connective tissue elements were of normal size and shape with no nuclear abnormality. In cases with severe cellular pleomorphism most cell forms were wildly irregular and many giant multinucleate forms were visible. Slight and moderate cellular pleomorphism varied between the two extremes. The degree of cellular pleomorphism was compared with the long-term outcome after surgery. The result of this comparison showed no obvious significant difference between the degree of cellular pleomorphism and the prognosis after lobectomy $(P > 0.5)$.

(ii) Presence of mitoses. A thorough search of all available histological material of the 49 Alien tissue cases failed to reveal a single mitotic figure in any of the sections examined.

(iii) Calcification of tissue. Calcification of tissue within the Alien tissue lesion was noted in nineteen of the forty-nine cases (39 per cent). The post-operative results in these 19 cases were compared with the remaining Alien tissue patients in Tables 16 and 17a and b. From these it will be seen that the patients who had a partly calcified Alien tissue abnormality fared significantly better than the remaining patients in the Alien tissue group $(P < 0.05$ for fits and $P < 0.5$ for personality and social adjustment).

(iv) Abnormal vascular proliferation. Abnormal vascular proliferation was a microscopic feature in 19 of the 49 Alien tissue lesions (39 per cent). By definition it was an essential criterion in the four patients with 'vascular' abnormalities but it was also seen in five patients with an Astrocytic glial lesion, six patients with a mixed glial lesion and four patients with a neuronoglial (ganglioglial) lesion. The presence of abnormal vascular proliferation was compared with the long-term outcome after surgery but showed no obvious significant correlation with the post-operative prognosis.

(v) Tissue necrosis. Tissue necrosis was visible in only three (6 per cent) of the 49 Alien tissue lesions, too few to assess its significance, if any, on the long-term prognosis after surgery.

(vi) Microcyst formation. The final histological variable to be assessed within the Alien tissue group concerned the presence of cystic degeneration in the temporal lobe lesions. In fact, microcyst formation was seen in 20 of the 49 Alien tissue abnormalities (41 per cent). Its presence was compared with the eventual outcome after surgery and showed no obvious correlation with the post-operative prognosis.

Alien tissue subgroups: neoplasm or maldevelopment. The present in-

Table 16. *Results of surgery in patients with calcification within their Alien tissue lesion*

Diagnostic category	Case No.	Sex	Length of follow-up (yrs)	Effect of surgery on fits	Effect of surgery on personality and social adjustment	Comments
Oligodendrocytic glial lesion	103	F	15	Worse	Unaltered	Died. Recurrence of lesion
Mixed glial lesion	69	M	11	Improved	Normal life	
	104	F	14	Fit-free	Normal life	
	133	F	20	Fit-free	Normal life	
	153	M	10	Fit-free	Normal life	
	164	M	2	Fit-free	Normal life	
	181	M	12	Fit-free	Normal life	
	197	M	1	Fit-free	Normal life	
	207	F	5	Fit-free	Normal life	
	208	F	22	Fit-free	Worse	Now schizophrenic
Neuronoglial lesion (ganglioglial)	7	M	2	Fit-free	Normal life	
	10	M	2	Fit-free	Worse	Aggressive and unmanageable
	102	F	14	Fit-free	Worse	Schizophrenic
	144	M	14	Fit-free	Worse	Schizophrenic – committed suicide
	162	M	15	Fit-free	Normal life	
	230	M	2	Worse	Worse	Aggressive. Behaviour problem
Vascular lesion	30	M	12	Improved	Unaltered	
	32	M	2	Fit-free	Worse	Died. Suicide
	188	F	3	Improved	Improved	

Table 17a. *Effect of surgery on fits*

	No. of patients	Fit-free or improved	Unaltered or worse
Patients with calcified Alien tissue lesions	19	17 (89%)	2 (11%)
Remaining Alien tissue patients	29 (one patient no follow-up)	20 (69%)	9 (31%)

Patients with calcified lesions had more chance of improvement in their fit pattern, $P < 0.05$

Table 17b. *Effect of surgery on personality and social adjustment*

	No. of patients	Normal life or improved life	Unaltered or worse
Patients with calcified Alien tissue lesions	19	12 (63%)	7 (37%)
Remaining Alien tissue patients	29	15 (52%)	14 (48%)

Patients with calcified lesions had slightly more chance of improved social adjustment, $P < 0.5$

vestigation concerns a small number of discrete abnormalities in one lobe of the brain. Yet it undoubtedly underlines many of the difficulties in differentiation between 'neoplasm' and 'maldevelopment'. Nevertheless, the classification of lesions into 'monoglial', 'mixed glial', 'neuronoglial' and 'vascular' has served to uncover some differences which may have future clinical use. In particular, the evidence suggests that the monoglial lesions (both the astrocytic and the oligodendrocytic) are true neoplasms and that the microscopic assessment of 'complete removal' is the only significant indicator of a likely recurrence. On the other hand, the mixed glial lesions (astrocytic *plus* oligodendrocytic), the neuronoglial lesions, and the vascular lesions, in the temporal lobe at least, appear to be maldevelopmental.

The evidence also shows that patients with the mixed glial lesions and the ganglioglial type of neuronoglial lesion improved significantly in their subsequent fit rate after lobectomy and that calcification within an Alien tissue lesion was also a good prognostic sign.

Group 4.   Ammon's horn sclerosis

Ammon's horn or hippocampal sclerosis is by far the commonest temporal lobectomy lesion. In the present series, 122 patients (49.3 per cent) had a sclerotic Ammon's horn. They consisted of 107 cases (43 per cent) in whom the sclerotic Ammon's horn was the only abnormality in their resected temporal lobe, and a further 15 from the 18 patients in the Double pathology group. The results from the Double pathology group differ in certain respects from those with a single lesion and are discussed later.

Perhaps because Ammon's horn sclerosis is the commonest lobectomy lesion, it has excited the greatest research interest since its discovery at the, naked-eye level by Bouchet and Cazauvieilh in 1825. In turn, Sommer (1880), who first defined it histologically, Hughlings Jackson and Coleman (1898), Turner J. (1907), Spielmeyer (1927), Scholz (1933) and many others have used their talents to establish the role of hippocampal sclerosis in epilepsy. More recently, however, the neuropathological contributions of Corsellis (1970a & b) have been unmatched. Moreover, the classical approach of neuropathology has been advanced by the development of experiments involving seizure production in animals (Meldrum & Brierley, 1973; Meldrum, 1975, 1976, 1981, 1983), and from all these sources the current view is that the initial neuronal damage in the hippocampus, as well as in the other vulnerable areas, is linked closely to the metabolic and ionic events arising during the greatly enhanced neuronal activity of a seizure. The consequent glial reaction and eventual scarring gradually 'ripen' (Earle, Baldwin & Penfield, 1953) and sooner or later may disrupt normal cerebral activity with the induction of further epileptic attacks.

Histologically, the term 'Ammon's horn sclerosis' is used to identify a patterned loss of nerve cells in the hippocampus with accompanying fibrous gliosis and a variable degree of shrinkage and atrophy. However, the degree of nerve-cell loss varies from case to case and in the present survey three distinct types of damage were seen. Two of the three have been named previously (Margerison & Corsellis, 1966); the first, and commonest, was termed 'Classical' Ammon's horn sclerosis and in this variety the hippocampal nerve-cell loss is most severe in the Sommer sector (H1) and in the end folium (H3–5). The second, and rarer, lesion involved only the end folium and is termed end folium sclerosis. However, in many patients the hippocampal damage is so severe that there is an almost complete loss of hippocampal neurons; for convenience this has been termed 'Total' Ammon's horn sclerosis.

The possibility that the various types of hippocampal damage might relate to the severity of the patient's epilepsy or to some other clinical variable was also considered. In order to test this hypothesis, the cases were accordingly subdivided into the three histological types. In fact, the results show that 57 per cent of patients had a Classical Ammon's horn sclerosis, 39 per cent had a Total Ammon's horn sclerosis, and 4 per cent had an end folium sclerosis. In addition, there was definite histological evidence in every case that the sclerotic damage extended to some degree beyond the confines of the hippocampus and this was signified by gliosis in the adjacent temporal lobe white matter. Particular note was also taken of any cortical nerve-cell damage in the adjacent temporal gyri, which occurred in 27 per cent of patients, and also of amygdaloid damage, which was visible in 76 per cent. Nevertheless, when the various lesions were correlated with the complete clinical data, there was no apparent correlation between any of them and the clinical history. It would appear, therefore, that the mere presence of hippocampal damage occurring in early life, rather than its type and severity, is more important in the production of further epileptogenic activity.

The post-operative results in the Ammon's horn sclerosis group reinforce much previously reported data (Falconer, Hill, Meyer, Mitchell & Pond, 1955; Kennedy & Hill, 1958; Taylor & Falconer, 1968; Taylor, 1972), yet a great deal of information concerning the later lobectomy patients has never been published, and the accumulation of these more recent data has uncovered several new relationships and clarified several others.

First, no less than 81 per cent of the group suffered some form of 'cerebral insult', which may have contributed towards the onset of their temporal lobe epilepsy. Indeed, 18 per cent had more than one possible predisposing factor. The most common and well-documented 'cerebral insult' was the history of febrile convulsions in infancy (Falconer, Serafetinides & Corsellis, 1964). This was found in 50 patients and was highly significant ($P < 0.0001$).

Less expected, however, was a moderately significant association between Ammon's horn sclerosis and birth injury (19 patients, $P < 0.02$). This had been claimed previously but not confirmed (Earle, Baldwin & Penfield, 1953). The significance of the association, however, does not necessarily imply that the causative mechanisms were as described in the Canadian paper or that birth injury is a major factor in the production of Ammon's horn sclerosis. A third correlation was also confirmed in the present material. This was between Ammon's horn sclerosis and a previous history of status epilepticus ($P < 0.02$). However, the apparent association between the last two features may be more doubtful than supposed.

The post-operative results from the present series, however, are quite clear. The operation produced either a dramatic reduction or a total abolition of fits in 80 per cent of patients after an average follow-up assessment of eight years ($P < 0.0001$). The effect of operation on personality and social adjustment was also good, with a significant chance of improvement at the level $P < 0.001$. Previous studies have shown the value of lobectomy in patients where the excised specimen contained a 'definite lesion' (Falconer, Serafetinides & Corsellis, 1964) and where the lesion is not only 'specific' but 'circumscribed' (Jensen & Klinken, 1976). However, no other clinico-pathological study has contained sufficient patients for such a dramatic association to be demonstrated between lobectomy results and a single neuropathological entity.

In summary, therefore, the Ammon's horn sclerosis group is the largest of the series (43 per cent), with the youngest mean age at first fit (mean age 5.19 years). It is significantly associated with a history of febrile convulsions, birth injury, and episodes of status epilepticus. The postoperative results give a dramatic and significant chance of improvement in both fit frequency and later adjustment to life and appear to be highly encouraging.

Group 5.   Inflammatory lesions

There were 11 patients (4.4 per cent of the series), each with evidence of an inflammatory process in the resected lobe. In addition three of these (Case Nos. 15, 16, and 48) had a sclerotic Ammon's horn and were classified in the Double pathology group.

The group diagnosis was made on histological appearances but, not surprisingly, a high proportion (nine cases) had suffered from a confirmed cerebral infection before the onset of their fits but in no case had a causative organism been identified. Four patients (Case Nos. 16, 62, 83, and 224) had a history of mastoid ear infection complicated by cerebral abscess, four others (Case Nos. 15, 48, 193 and 249) had had a previous episode of meningitis, and one patient (Case No. 130) had encephalitis with convulsions. Of the two patients without confirmed infection, Case No. 247 developed frequent 'idiopathic' seizures with aggressive outbursts when aged five years. Case No. 214 developed fits when aged 18 years; she had a raised CSF protein and a high ESR but the exact diagnosis was never established. The pathology in these two cases was that of a 'burnt out' encephalitis and a 'smouldering' leptomeningitis respectively.

In fact, the neuropathological features of all patients mirrored their clinical presentations, i.e. a healed cerebral abscess (four cases), a 'burnt out' or 'smouldering' leptomeningitis (five cases) or a 'quiescent' encephalitis (two cases). The type of inflammatory cell response also varied from patient to patient; some showed an infiltration composed of a mixture of polymorphs and lymphocytes, whereas others had only lymphocytes. As expected, the cases of meningitis and encephalitis showed widespread damage throughout the lobe to the very edge of the resection; in this context it is interesting to note that in one case (Case No. 247), where the whole brain has since been studied, the encephalitic process virtually destroyed the remainder of the left hemisphere but had largely spared the right.

On the other hand, the cerebral abscesses were relatively circumscribed and in all four patients the damage was limited, histologically, to the middle temporal, inferior temporal, and the fusiform gyri. It was considered that these latter lesions had been completely resected at operation.

Direct comparison between the inflammatory lesions of the present series and those from other lobectomy studies is hindered by the previous tendency to classify pathology into either Focal or Discrete lesions or Diffuse and Disseminated lesions (see Falconer, Serafetinides & Corsellis, 1964, for discussion). For example, Jensen and Klinken (1976) classify their Case No. 4 (toxoplasmic meningo-encephalitis) as a calcified focal lesion in their category of 'Focal Tumours and well-defined non-neoplastic lesions' (Group 1), whereas most other cerebral infections appear in Group 5 (Perivascular lymphocytic and histiocytic infiltration cases). Nevertheless, 24 per cent of their 74 patients had a history of cerebral infection and the only positive clinico-pathological correlation in their series was a clinical history cf cerebral infection and the occurrence of 'perivascular infiltration', in the resected lobe. A different choice of pathological classification may well have given much more relevant information to augment the massive clinical review of Jensen (1975a, b, c, 1976a, b, c). Despite this, however, it is clear that the incidence of 24 per cent in Jensen's series is much greater than the 4.4 per cent of the present study; the differences are presumably due to patient selection rather than to an overall difference in incidence of temporal lobe infection.

In the present series, the inflammatory group gave rise to epilepsy at an early age (mean age 8.6 years) reflecting the higher incidence of cerebral infection in young children (*Registrar General's Statistical Review of England and Wales*, 1972). The post-operative results show no overall alteration in fit frequency or social adjustment, which may result from the small numbers in the group and also the variable nature of the pathology, whereas one might have expected worse results from the widespread infections and better results from the more localized ones.

Group 6.   Indefinite pathology
The histological appearances in the 25 members (10 per cent of the series) were some of the most difficult to interpret. Indeed, the only reason for placing them together was the singular difficulty in deciding, in each case, whether the lobe was abnormal. However, it was concluded that their microscopic appearances lay in the borderland between the normal and the abnormal lobe, and they were placed accordingly in the 'indefinite' pathology category. Nevertheless, it soon became apparent that the lesions clustered into certain subgroups, in that 17 lobes (68 per cent of

the group) showed an unusual degree of white matter gliosis with no discernible cortical nerve cell loss, and four others (16 per cent) had small numbers of large, bizarre cells scattered in an otherwise abnormal amygdaloid nucleus. The remainder (four cases) showed microscopic appearances which were probably abnormal but were too indefinite to diagnose with confidence.

Of the 17 cases with an unusual degree of gliosis, no less than 10 had been incompletely resected and one or more parts of the temporal lobe were unavailable for examination. It is a matter of speculation, therefore, whether or not the missing areas contained any definite pathology, and in this context it is interesting that five of these seventeen patients had had a previous head injury and that there was a significant association between past head injury and the group as a whole at the level $P < 0.01$.

The four patients with unusual glia in the amygdaloid nucleus represent a fascinating rarity. The pertinent histological feature was the presence of small collections of unusually large hyperchromatic glial cells, resembling giant astrocytes, in the amygdaloid nucleus. There was no evidence of disruption of the amygdaloid cytoarchitecture and no mitoses. It was difficult to determine whether they represented a normal variation of amygdaloid cytoarchitecture or perhaps some minute glial malformation.

The remaining four patients showed unusual perivascular cuffing of vessels in the roof of the inferior horn (Case No. 111), very recent cortical and white matter damage in the inferior temporal gyrus adjacent to the line of recent operative haemorrhage (Case No. 23), unusually dense fibrous thickening of the leptomeninges with a few haemosiderin-containing macrophages beneath the thickened meninges (Case No. 50), and Case No. 223 where there were a few haemosiderin-containing macrophages surrounding several vessels in the inferior temporal gyrus.

Other lobectomy studies have considered patients with 'indefinite' or 'equivocal' pathology (see Jensen & Klinken, 1976, for detailed references). The incidence varies from 0 per cent to 58 per cent, according to the survey studied, yet there have been no definite conclusions. Falconer, Serafetinides, and Corsellis (1964) noted that most cases exhibited some degree of subpial or marginal gliosis and that many showed a variable degree of white matter gliosis. However, they quote Crome (1955) in stating that, at least in post-mortem material, the damage is too variable, too common, and too ill-understood to be interpreted as a definite abnormality.

Jensen and Klinken (1976) consider that the notion of 'equivocal' change is a challenge to the neuropathologist as well as to the clinician.

In the present study, the Indefinite pathology group began to have epileptic fits in adolescence or early adult life (mean age 14.72 years). The post-operative results show that while there was no alteration in fit frequency, the psychosocial adjustment to life is significantly worse ($P < 0.01$). However, despite the group results, it is interesting to note that the four patients with unusual glia in the amygdaloid all benefited from operation. Nevertheless, the overall effect of lobectomy in the group would appear to have been harmful. In addition, the average age at first fit, the significant association with previous head injury, and the poor post-operative outcome are all reminiscent of the findings in the Trauma group, suggesting perhaps that some members of the Indefinite group may have a 'traumatic' aetiology. The most likely candidates would appear to be those with undue gliosis of the lobe and it may be that certain of these cases had shown the effects of a previous head injury.

In summary, therefore, the Indefinite pathology group represents some 10 per cent of the present series. Most of the group show an unusual degree of white matter gliosis, and there are certain statistical similarities between the group and the Group 2 Trauma category. In addition, a few patients show an unusual glial presence in an otherwise normal amygdaloid nucleus, and these cases have benefited from operation, whereas the group as a whole did not. These latter cases may possibly represent a minute glial abnormality.

Group 7.   No apparent abnormality
This category contains all patients whose lobe appeared completely normal both on naked-eye and microscopical examination. It consists of 41 patients (16.2 per cent) and is the second largest in the series.

The problem of the 'normal temporal lobe' has been considered by other workers, often in association with 'equivocal' or 'indefinite' pathology (Falconer, Serafetinides & Corsellis, 1964; Green & Scheetz, 1964; Corsellis, 1970a; Jensen & Klinken, 1976). Corsellis (1970a) summarized the situation when he stated 'No definite structural abnormality can be found in roughly one in five specimens. At times this is probably due to the simple fact that none is present, but other possibilities have to be considered'. He then proposed the possibility that in certain cases the pre-operative lateralization was faulty and that the opposite temporal lobe contained the lesion. He also considered the known cases where temporal lobe epilepsy had occurred in the presence of a lesion outside the temporal lobe (Falconer, Driver & Serafetinides, 1962).

Green and Scheetz (1964) found an incidence of 17.9 per cent of 'no demonstrable pathology' in their 78 cases, but Jensen and Klinken (1976) had only three cases of 'no structural abnormality' in their series of 74. In the members of the present group, epilepsy began in early adult life (mean age 15.37 years) and the post-operative results were uniformly bad. After operation, the average fit frequency was not significantly altered, but the social or personal outcome was much worse ($P < 0.005$). As suggested by Corsellis (1970a), one explanation for these poor results might be that a distant cerebral lesion had been missed by the surgeon, or perhaps that there was no structural abnormality in the brain at all. However, if this were so, it might seem reasonable to expect either no significant change in both the fit rate and the psychosocial adjustment, or perhaps a uniform deterioration in both, but the actual findings of an unaltered fit rate and a great deterioration in psychosocial adjustment are not easy to understand unless, as increasingly suspected, the resected areas have a special role to play in the more complex aspects of human behaviour.

Before operation, five patients in the group were considered to have been psychotic, six people had been considered to be excessively violent and one woman had recurrent bouts of depression. This number of disturbed patients is slightly higher than in any other diagnostic group and may go some way to explain the results, but after operation not only did the psychotic patients remain unchanged, one other became schizophrenic. Only one of the six aggressive patients improved and three others became violent for the first time. In addition, nine patients developed recurrent bouts of depression. Two patients developed serious, permanent physical handicaps and no fewer than five of the group have died. Three people died in a fit or in a bout of status epilepticus, one person committed suicide, and one died from a cause unrelated to the lobectomy.

This catalogue of disaster is not seen in such florid form in any other group, and although it may be considered coincidental, it may well indicate that to remove a normal temporal lobe in a patient already plagued by intractable drug-resistant epilepsy can only result in a deterioration of the already difficult situation.

Group 8.   Double pathology lesions
The last group in the series was chosen, not only because its 18 members (7.2 per cent of the series) had two distinct abnormalities, but also to test the hypothesis that the presence of these two separate lesions might influence the clinical history and the eventual outcome after surgery. An examination of the 18 cases showed two subgroups; fifteen patients with an Ammon's horn sclerosis as one part of the dual pathology and three patients each with a large developmental cyst in association with an Alien tissue lesion. An examination of the results showed certain features which suggested that the presence of a second lesion does modify the clinical presentation and also the post-operative outcome. First, a study of the 15 Double pathology Ammon's horn sclerotics revealed a slightly later mean age at first fit when compared with the 'pure' Ammon's horn sclerotics (mean age 8.24 compared with 5.19 years). Secondly, only one of the Double pathology group had had a past history of febrile convulsions in infancy, as compared with 50 of the 107 patients with the single Ammon's horn lesion.

Furthermore, 27 per cent of patients with Double pathology had a history of status epilepticus, as compared with 15 per cent in the single lesion category. However, the most striking differences were seen in the results after lobectomy. In the 'pure' Ammon's horn sclerosis group, the post-operative fit frequency and social adjustment were significantly improved but in the Double Pathology lesions, the fit frequency was not statistically altered and the effect on personality and social adjustment was disastrous; only five patients were improved, whereas ten were unaltered or worse. Of these ten patients, three became severely depressed, two became schizophrenic, one person became aggressive and unmanageable, and two had permanent post-operative physical handicaps. The greatly differing results may simply reflect the smaller number of patients in the Double pathology Ammon's horn group. However, a more likely explanation is that the presence of the second lesion does modify the clinical response; the second lesion was either an inflammatory process, a cortical scar, or an Alien tissue lesion, and from previous results it has been seen that the Inflammatory lesions and the Trauma group have a poor post-operative outcome. In addition, the two Double pathology patients who became schizophrenic had a ganglioglial lesion as their second pathology and the ganglioglial patients tended to have a psychiatrically poor post-operative course. Thus it would appear that patients with a second lesion in combination with an Ammon's horn sclerosis, mimic the post-operative behaviour of the second lesion rather than respond as patients with a 'pure' Ammon's horn lesion.

The three remaining Double pathology patients (Case Nos. 98, 137, and 153) are too few to assess. Each had an Alien tissue lesion combined with a large ependymal-lined 'developmental' cyst. The Alien tissue abnormality in Case No. 98 was a ganglioglial lesion but there was no follow-up information, as the patient disappeared without trace. In patients Nos. 137 and 153, the Alien tissue lesion was a mixed glial abnormality, and both patients are fit-free and completely well some five and ten years after operation respectively.

Double pathology lobectomies have been catalogued previously (Falconer, Serafetinides & Corsellis, 1964), but in no study has a separate Double pathology group been investigated. The results from the present study go some way to suggest that the presence of two abnormalities does modify the clinical presentation and the post-operative outcome, and in some cases when one of the lesions is a sclerotic Ammon's horn, the post-operative behaviour seems related more to the second lesion than to the hippocampal pathology. In future material it may be justified, therefore, to classify such cases within the groupings of the second lesion to give a more valid prediction of the post-operative behaviour.

4. Conclusions: assessment of clinico-pathological results

'LEAGUE TABLE OF BENEFIT FROM SURGERY'

The preceding chapters contain a review of all available cases of *en bloc* resection of the temporal lobe performed by Mr. Murray Falconer during the 25 years beginning in January 1950.

During the study a modified system of neuropathological classification was used, and from this it has been possible, for the first time, to provide a detailed guide to the long-term results of surgery as they vary with the different types of temporal lobe pathology. This guide, which I have termed a 'League table of benefit from surgery', does not seriously conflict with previously available information (Falconer, Serafetinides & Corsellis, 1964; Jensen & Klinkén, 1976) but enlarges its scope.

The league table is detailed in Table 18; it shows that the Ammon's horn sclerosis patients are most likely to benefit significantly, with a reduction or complete abolition of fits and a marked improvement in their social adjustment to life. These patients form nearly 50 per cent of the whole series, and the value of surgery in their treatment would not appear to be in doubt. Within the Ammon's horn sclerosis group, the close association with a previous episode of febrile convulsions is underlined, and for the first time a statistically significant association with birth injury was confirmed.

The league table of benefit shows two other categories with a significant reduction in their post-operative fit rate, but with no significant alteration in post-operative personality and social adjustment to life. These two are the mixed glial and the ganglioglial malformations, microscopically similar apart from the presence of abnormal nerve cells in the latter lesion. At first sight both groups would appear to deserve equal scrutiny by the neurosurgeons but the problem, however, is not so straightforward in that they each contained four patients with Double pathology, and if these dual pathology patients are considered, together with their appropriate mixed glial or ganglioglial class, a dramatic difference is seen. Thus, the mixed glial category continues to do very well, both in reduction of seizure rate as well as social adjustment to life, whereas the ganglioglial patients become fit-free but are prone to the most disastrous psychiatric disturbances. Four of the nine ganglioglial

Table 18. *Temporal lobectomy series: 249 patients. Effects of surgery: league table of benefit*

	Diagnostic groups	No. of patients in group	% of total sample	Comments
(1)	Ammon's horn sclerosis	107	43.0	Benefit: both fit frequency and social adjustment
(2)	Mixed glial	9	3.6	Benefit: fits only. Social adjustment unaffected
	Neuronoglial (ganglioglial)	5	3.0	Benefit; fits only. Social adjustment unaffected
(3)	Astrocytic	8	3.2	Unaffected
	Oligodendrocytic	5	2.0	Unaffected
	Neuronoglial (cortical dysplasia)	8	3.2	Unaffected
	Vascular	3	1.2	Unaffected
	Developmental lesion	5	2.0	Unaffected
	Inflammatory	8	3.2	Unaffected
	Double pathology	18	7.3	Unaffected
(4)	Trauma	7	2.8	Fits unaffected. Social adjustment worse
	Indefinite pathology	25	10.0	Fits unaffected. Social adjustment worse
	No apparent abnormality	41	16.5	Fits unaffected. Social adjustment worse

patients became schizophrenic after lobectomy, and two were aggressive and unmanageable. Adequate explanations for these differences are unclear, but it would appear to be potentially harmful to operate on the ganglioglial subgroup and beneficial to remove the mixed glial ones.

Most of the remaining groups remain apparently unaltered by operation, both in their fit frequency and social adjustment to life. Thus, the Double pathology patients, nearly all of whom have a sclerotic Ammon's horn as one part of their temporal lobe damage, do not share the same good prognosis of the single lesion Ammon's horn group. Their post-operative outcome tends to follow the characteristic behaviour expected from the second lesion and it would seem prudent to reclassify these cases accordingly.

The astrocytic glial and the oligodendrocytic glial lesions are also unaffected statistically by lobectomy. They give rise to late-onset epilepsy and behave as very slowly growing neoplasms rather than malformations. In addition, specimens which were considered to have been incompletely resected at operation were almost certain eventually to recur. Indeed, patients whose temporal lobe pathology report suggested an incompletely resected lesion fared significantly worse both in fit frequency and post-operative adjustment to life, as compared with other patients in the series.

Three other groups showed no significant post-operative alteration in fit rate and social adjustment to life. These were the vascular malformations (4 cases), the cortical dysplasia type of neuronoglial malformation (8 cases) and the inflammatory lesions (11 cases). Of these, the inflammatory group was the largest and there was a positive history of cerebral infection in nine.

The inflammatory lesions give rise to early-onset epilepsy and would appear to be easily diagnosed before operation. Patients with a generalized leptomeningitis or an encephalitis are most likely to have pathology spreading beyond the confines of the resected temporal lobe and are unlikely to be helped by surgery. However, patients with a temporal lobe abscess have more localized pathology and their fits may possibly be controlled or improved by operation.

Patients with the cortical dysplasia type of lesion have become the focus of much recent investigation (personal communications from Professor David Taylor and Dr. I. Janota), and it is hoped that with a larger number of cases, more definitive information on the results of surgery will be obtained.

Finally, the league table of benefit shows three groups where the neurosurgical results reveal an unaltered fit pattern but a significant deterioration in the personality and social adjustment to life. These are the Trauma group, the Indefinite pathology group, and the No apparent abnormality group. The Trauma group, almost without exception, had focal scarring with widespread white matter gliosis, often with visible demyelination of nerve fibres, spreading to the limits of the resected lobe. It is reasonable to suppose that most of these patients had damage in adjacent parts of the unresected brain, and it is not surprising that lobectomy did not improve their symptoms. Similarly, nearly 70 per cent of the Indefinite pathology group had an abnormal degree of gliosis throughout the resected lobe and many had a past history of head injury.

In their case also, the spread of pathology to the edge of the resected specimen is a bad prognostic sign.

The 'No apparent abnormality' group formed 16 per cent of the series. The post-operative catalogue of epileptic, psychiatric, and physical disasters is not seen in any other group and is not easy to explain. It may be that an adjacent lesion, or an abnormality in the opposite temporal lobe had been missed, or perhaps the brain showed no structural abnormality at all. Nevertheless, the results do suggest that to remove a normal temporal lobe in a patient crippled by drug-resistant temporal lobe epilepsy may do more harm than good.

Taken together the results suggest that the operation of anterior temporal lobectomy does indeed have a place in the successful treatment of severe temporal lobe epilepsy, most particularly in those patients with an Ammon's horn sclerosis.

References

Adams, J. Hume. (1984). Head injury. In *Greenfield's Neuropathology*, 4th edn. (eds. Adams, J. Hume, Corsellis, J. A. N. & Duchen, L. W.), Chap. 3, pp. 85–124. Arnold, London.

Bailey, P. & Bucy, P. C. (1929). Oligodendrogliomas of the brain. *J. Pathol. Bacteriol.* **32**, 735–51.

—— & Gibbs, F. A. (1951). The surgical treatment of psycho-motor epilepsy. *J. Amer. Med. Assoc.* **145**, 365–70.

Bancroft, J. D. & Stevens, A. (1982). *Theory and practice of histological techniques,* 2nd edn. Churchill Livingstone, Edinburgh and London.

Barraclough, B. (1981). Suicide and epilepsy. In *Psychiatry and epilepsy* (eds. Reynolds, E. H. & Trimble, M. R.). Churchill Livingstone, Edinburgh and London.

Bouchet, C. & Cazauvieilh (1825). De l'épilepsie considérée dans ses rapports avec l'aliénation mentale. Recherches sur la nature et le siège de ces deux maladies. *Arch. gén. méd., (Paris)*, **9**, 510–42.

Bruton, C. J. (1984). The pathology of temporal lobectomy. *MD Thesis (London University)*.

Carter, C. O., David, P. A & Laurence, K. M. (1968). A family study of major central nervous system malformations in South Wales. *J. Med. Genet.* **5**, 81–106.

Cavanagh, J. B. (1958). On certain small tumours encountered in the temporal lobe. *Brain*, **81**, 389–405.

—— & Meyer, A. (1956). Aetiological aspects of Ammon's horn sclerosis associated with temporal lobe epilepsy. *Brit. Med. J.,* **2**, 1403–7.

Corsellis, J. A. N. (1970a). The neuropathology of temporal lobe epilepsy. In *Modern trends in neurology*, No. 6, (ed. Williams D.) pp. 254–70. Butterworth, London.

—— (1970b). The pathological anatomy of the temporal lobe with special reference to the limbic areas. In *Modern trends in psychological medicine*, No. 2, (ed. Price, J. H.), pp. 296–325. Butterworth, London.

—— & Bruton, C. J. (1983). Neuropathology of status epilepticus in humans. In *Advances in neurology*, No. 34, *Status epilepticus mechanism of brain damage and treatment*, (eds. Delgado-Escueta, A. V., Wasterlain, C. G., Treiman, D. M. & Porter, R. J.), pp. 129–40. Raven Press, New York.

—— & Meldrum, B. S. (1984). Epilepsy. In *Greenfield's Neuropathology*, 4th edn., chap. 9 (eds. Hume Adams J., Corsellis, J. A. N. & Duchen, L. W.) pp. 921–50. Arnold, London.

Courville, C. B. (1930). Ganglioglioma; tumour of the nervous system. A review of the literature and a report of two cases. *Arch. Neurol. Psychiat. (Chicago)*, **24**, 439–91.

—— (1957) Traumatic lesions of the temporal lobe as an essential cause of psychomotor epilepsy. In *Temporal lobe epilepsy* (eds. Baldwin, M. & Bailey, P.) pp. 220–39. Charles C. Thomas, Illinois, USA.

Crome, L. (1955). A morphological critique of temporal lobectomy. *Lancet*, 1, 882–4.

——& Stern, J. (1972). *The pathology of mental retardation*, 2nd edn. Churchill Livingstone, Edinburgh and London.

del Rio Hortega, P. (1919). El'tercer elemento' de los centros nerviosos. *Bol. Soc. esp. Biol.*, 9, 69–120.

—— (1921). Estudios sobre la neuroglia. La glia de escasas radiaciones (oligodendroglia). *Bol. Real. Soc. esp. Hist. Nat.*, 21, 63–92.

Earle, K. M., Baldwin, M. & Penfield, W. (1953). Incisural sclerosis and temporal lobe seizures produced by hippocampal herniation at birth. *Arch. Neurol. Psychiat. (Chicago)*, 69, 27–42.

Edgar, R. & Baldwin, M. (1960). Vascular malformations associated with temporal lobe epilepsy. *J. Neurosurg.* 17, 638–56.

Elizan, T. S. & Fabiyi, A. (1970). Congenital and neonatal anomalies linked with viral infections in experimental animals. *Amer. J. Obstet. Gynaecol.*, 106, 147–65.

Eng, L. F. & DeArmond, S. J. (1982). Immunocytochemical studies of astrocytes in normal development and disease. In *Advances in cellular neurobiology, No. 3.* (eds. Fedoross, S. & Hertz, L.) Academic Press Inc., USA.

Esquirol, E. (1838). *Des maladies mentales-médicales, hygiéniques et médicolégales*, 1, pp. 274–336. Ballière, Paris.

Falconer, M. A. (1965). The surgical treatment of temporal lobe epilepsy. *Neurochirurg.*, 8, 160–72.

—— (1968). The significance of mesial temporal sclerosis in epilepsy. *Guy's Hosp. Reports*, 117, 1–12.

—— (1969). Temporal lobe epilepsy in childhood and adolescence with reference to surgical treatment. *6th Wilder Penfield Lecture*, Hosp. Pediatría, Mexico City, October, 1969.

—— & Serafetinides, E. A. (1963). A follow-up study of surgery in temporal lobe epilepsy. *J. Neurol. Neurosurg. Psychiat*, 26, 154–65.

—— & Taylor, D. C. (1968). Surgical treatment of drug resistant epilepsy due to mesial temporal sclerosis: etiology and significance. *Arch. Neurol. (Chicago)*, 19, 353–61.

——, Driver, M. V. & Serafetinides, E. A. (1962). Temporal lobe epilepsy due to distant lesions: two cases relieved by operation. *Brain*, 85, 521–34.

——, Serafetinides, E. A. & Corsellis, J. A. N. (1964). Etiology and pathogenesis of temporal lobe epilepsy. *Arch. Neurol. (Chicago)*, 10, 233–48.

——, Pond, D. A., Meyer, A. & Woolf, A. L. (1953). Temporal lobe epilepsy with personality and behavioural disorders caused by an unusual calcifying lesion. *J. Neurol. Neurosurg. Psychiat*, 16, 234–44.

——, Hill, D., Meyer, A., Mitchell, W. & Pond, D. A. (1955). Treatment of temporal lobe epilepsy by temporal lobectomy: a survey of findings and results. *Lancet*, 1, 827–35.

Falret, J. (1860). De l'état mental des épileptiques. *Arch. gén. méd.*, **16**, 661–79. P. Asselin, Paris.

Gastaut, H. (1959). Etiology, pathology and pathogenesis of temporal lobe epilepsy. *Epilepsy News Letter No. 15 (International League Against Epilepsy)*, pp. 15–24.

Gibbs, F. A., Gibbs, E. L. & Lennox, W. G. (1937). Epilepsy: a paroxysmal cerebral dysrhythmia. *Brain*, **60**, 377–88.

Goddard, G. V. (1964). Functions of the amygdala. *Psychol. Bull.* **62**, 89–109.

Gowers, Sir W. (1901). *Epilepsy and other chronic convulsive diseases, their causes, symptoms and treatment*, 2nd edn. Churchill, London.

Green, J. R. & Scheetz, D. G. (1964). Surgery of epileptogenic lesions of the temporal lobe. *Arch. Neurol. (Chicago)*, **10**, 135–48.

Griesinger, W. (1857). *Mental pathology and therapeutics.* (Trans. Lockhart Robertson & Rutherford.) New Sydenham Society, London.

Henriksen, P. B., Juul-Jensen, P. & Lund, M. (1970). The mortality of epileptics. In *Life assurance medicine* (ed. Brackenridge, R. D. C.), pp. 139–48. Pitman & Co., London.

Hicks, S. P. (1952). Symposium on cerebral palsy: some effects of ionising radiation and metabolic inhibition on developing mammalian nervous tissue. *J. Pediat.*, **40**, 489–513.

Hill, D. (1953). Discussion of surgery in temporal lobe epilepsy. *Proc. Roy. Soc. Med.*, **46**, 965–76.

—— Pond, D. A., Mitchell, W. & Falconer, M. A. (1957). Personality changes following temporal lobectomy for epilepsy. *J. Ment. Sci.* **103**, 18–27.

Holbourn, A. H. S. (1943). Mechanics of head injuries. *Lancet*, **2**, 438–41.

Jackson, J. H. (1875). On temporary mental disorders after epileptic paroxysms. In *Selected Writings of John Hughlings Jackson*, vol. 1. (ed. Taylor, J.), p. 124, Hodder and Stoughton (1931), London.

—— & Beevor, C. E. (1889). Case of a tumour of the right tempero-sphenoidal lobe bearing on the localisation of the sense of smell and the interpretation of a particular variety of epilepsy. *Brain*, **12**, 346–57.

—— & Coleman, W. S. (1898). Case of epilepsy with tasting movements and 'dreamy state': very small patch of softening in the left uncinate gyrus. *Brain*, **21**, 580–90.

Jakob, A. (1914). Zur Pathologie der Epilepsie. *Z. ges. Neurol. Psychiat.*, **23**, 1–65.

Jann Brown, W. (1973). Structural substrates of seizure foci in the human temporal lobe. *UCLA Forum Med. Sci.*, **17**, 339–74.

Jasper, H. & Kershman, J. (1941). Electroencephalographic classification of the epilepsies. *Arch. Neurol. Psychiat. (Chicago)*, **45**, 903–43.

—— Pertuisset, B. & Flanigin, H. (1951). Electroencephalographic and cortical electrograms in patients with temporal lobe seizures. *Arch. Neurol. Psychiat. (Chicago)*, **65**, 272–90.

Jennett, W. B. (1965). Predicting epilepsy after blunt head injury. *Brit. Med. J.* **1**, 1215–16.

Jensen, I. (1975(a)). Temporal lobe surgery around the world. Results, complications and mortality. *Acta neurol. Scand.*, **52**, 354–73.

—— (1975(b)). Temporal lobe epilepsy. Late mortality in patients treated with unilaterial temporal lobe resections. *Acta neurol. Scand.*, **52**, 374–80.

—— (1975(c)). Genetic factors in temporal lobe epilepsy. *Acta neurol. Scand.*, **52**, 381–94.

—— (1976(a)). Temporal lobe epilepsy. Etiological factors and surgical results. *Acta neurol. Scand.*, **53**, 103–18.

—— (1976(b)). Temporal lobe epilepsy. Types of seizure and surgical results. *Acta neurol. Scand.*, **53**, 335–57.

—— (1976(c)). Temporal lobe epilepsy. Social conditions and rehabilitation after surgery. *Acta neurol. Scand.*, **54**, 22–44.

—— & Klinken, L. (1976). Temporal lobe epilepsy and neuropathology: histological findings in resected temporal lobes correlated to surgical results and clinical aspects. *Acta neurol. Scand.*, **54**, 392–414.

—— & Larsen, J. K. (1979). Mental aspects of temporal lobe epilepsy. *J. Neurol. Neurosurg. Psychiat.*, **42**, 256–65.

Kalter, H. (1968). *Tetralogy of the central nervous system.* University of Chicago Press, Chicago, USA.

Kennedy, W. A. & Hill, D. (1958). The surgical prognostic significance of the electroencephalographic prediction of Ammon's horn sclerosis in epileptics. *J. Neurol. Neurosurg. Psychiat.*, **21**, 24–30.

Kernohan, J. W., Mabon, R. F., Svien, H. J. & Adson, A. W. (1949). Symposium on a new and simplified concept of gliomas. *Proc. Staff Meetings Mayo Clin.*, **24**, 71.

Kligman, D. & Goldberg, D. A. (1975). Temporal lobe epilepsy and aggression. *J. Nerv. Ment. Dis.*, **160**, 324–41.

Lennox, W. G. & Lennox, M. A. (1960). *Epilepsy and related disorders*, vols. 1 & 2. Churchill, London.

Lindenberg, R. (1971). Trauma of meninges and brain. In *Pathology of the nervous system*, vol. 2 (ed. Minckler, J.), pp. 1705–65. McGraw Hill, New York, USA.

Margerison, J. H. & Corsellis, J. A. N. (1966). Epilepsy and the temporal lobes: A clinical electroencephalographic and neuropathological study of the brain in epilepsy with particular reference to the temporal lobes. *Brain*, **89**, 499–530.

Mark, V. H. and Ervin, F. R. (1970). *Violence and the brain.* Harper and Row, New York.

Maspes, P. E. & Marossero, F. (1953). Survey of 28 patients operated for temporal lobe epilepsy. *Rev. neurol.*, **88**, 578–80.

Meldrum, B. S. (1975). Present views on hippocampal sclerosis and epilepsy. In *Modern trends in neurology*, No. 6 (ed. Williams, D.), pp. 223–39. Butterworths, London.

—— (1976). Secondary pathology of febrile and experimental convulsions. In *Brain dysfunction in infantile, febrile convulsions* (ed. Brazier, M. A. B. & Coceani, F.), pp. 213–22. Raven Press, New York.

—— (1981). Epilepsy. In *The molecular basis of neuropathology*, (eds. Davison, A. N. & Thompson, R. H. S.), pp. 265–301. Arnold, London.

—— (1983). Metabolic factors during prolonged seizures and their relation to nerve cell death. In *Neuropathology of status epilepticus in humans. Advances in* neurology, No. 34 (eds. Delgado-Escueta, A. V. Wasterlain, C. G., Treimann, D. M. & Porter, R. J.), pp. 261–75. Raven Press, New York.

—— & Brierley, J. B. (1973). Prolonged epileptic seizures in primates: ischaemic cell change and its relation to ictal physiological events. *Arch. Neurol. (Chicago)*, **28**, 10–17.

—— Vigouroux, R. A. & Brierley, J. B. (1973). Systemic factors and epileptic brain damage. *Arch. Neurol. (Chicago)*, **29**, 82–7.

Meyer, A., Falconer, M. A. & Beck, E. (1954). Pathological findings in temporal lobe epilepsy. *J. Neurol. Neurosurg. Psychiat.*, **17**, 276–85.

Millichap, J. G. (1968). *Febrile convulsions*. Macmillan, New York.

Nathaniel, E. J. H. & Nathaniel, D. R. (1981). The reactive astrocyte. In *Advances in cellular neurobiology*, vol. 2, pp. 249–301. (eds. Fedoross, S & Hertz, L.), Academic Press Inc., New York.

Nicholson, G. W. (1925). The nature of tumour formation. In *The Erasmus Wilson Lectures*. C.U.P., Cambridge.

Norman, R. M. (1963). Malformation of the nervous system, birth injury and diseases of early life. In *Greenfield's Neuropathology*, 2nd edn. (eds. Blackwood, W., McMenemey, W. H., Meyer, A., Norman, R. M. & Russell, D. S.), Chap. 6, pp. 324–440. Edward Arnold, London.

—— (1964). The neuropathology of status epilepticus. *Med. Sci. Law*, **4**, 46–51.

Ounsted, C. & Lindsay, J. (1981). The long term outcome of temporal lobe epilepsy in childhood. In *Psychiatry and epilepsy*, (eds. Reynolds, E. H. & Trimble, M. R.), Churchill Livingstone, Edinburgh & London.

——, —— & Norman, R. (1966). Biological factors in temporal lobe epilepsy. In *Clin. dev. med.*, No. 22. Wm. Heinemann, London.

Palay, S. L. (1966). The role of neuroglia in the organisation of the central nervous system. In *Nerve as a tissue* (eds. Rodahl, K. & Isskutz, B.), pp. 3–10. Harper (Hoeber), New York.

Pampiglione, G. & Kerridge, J. (1956). EEG abnormalities from the temporal lobes studied with sphenoidal electrodes. *J. Neurol. Neurosurg. Psychiat.*, **19**, 117–29.

Papez, J. W. (1937). 'A proposed mechanism of emotion'. *Arch. Neurol. Psychiat. (Chicago)*, **38**, 725–43.

Penfield, W. & Flanigin, H. (1950). Surgical therapy of temporal lobe seizures. *Arch. Neurol. Psychiat. (Chicago)*, **64**, 491–500.

——& Steelman, H. (1947). The treatment of focal epilepsy by cortical excision. *Ann. Surg.* **126**, 740–61.

—— & Ward, A. (1948). Calcifying epileptogenic lesions. *Arch. Neurol. Psychiat. (Chicago)*, **60**, 20–36.

Peters, A. & Palay, S. L. (1965). An electron microscope study of the distribution and patterns of astroglial processes in the central nervous system. *J. Anat.*, **99**, 419.

——, —— & Webster, H. de F. (1976). *The fine structure of the nervous system. The neurons and supporting cells*. Saunders, Philadelphia.

Pond, D. A. (1957). Psychiatric aspects of epilepsy. *J. Ind. Med. Prof.*, **3**, 1441–51.

——, Bidwell, B. H. & Stein, L. (1960). A survey of epilepsy in 14 General

Practices. 1. Demographic and medical data. *Psychiat. neurol. neurochirurg.*, **63**, 217–36.

Pudenz, R. H. & Sheldon, C. H. (1946). The lucite calvarium. A method for direct observation of the brain. II. Cranial trauma and brain motion. *J. Neurosurg.*, **3**, 487–505.

Ramón y Cajal, S. (1909). *Histologie du système nerveux de l'homme et des vertébrés.* Vols. 1–2 (trans: Dr. L. Azoulay.) Maloine, Paris.

—— (1913). Sobre un nuevo proceder de impregnación de la neuroglia y sus resultados en los centros nerviosos del hombre y animales. *Trab. Inst. Cajal invest. biol.,* **11**, 219–37.

—— (1916). El proceder del oro sublimado para la coloración de la neuroglia. *Trab. Lab. invest. biol., Univ. Madrid,* **14**, 155–62.

Rasmussen, T. (1969). The role of surgery in the treatment of focal epilepsy. *Clin. neurosurg.*, **16**, 288–314.

The Registrar General's *Statistical review of England and Wales for the Year 1972.* Part 1. HMSO, London.

Rey, J. H., Pond, D. A. & Evans, C. C. (1949). Clinical and electroencephalographic studies of temporal lobe function. *Proc. Roy. Med.*, **42**, 891–904.

Roberts, A. H. (1979). *Severe accidental head injury. An assessment of the longterm prognosis.* Macmillan, London.

Robertson, W. (1899). On a new method of obtaining a black reaction in certain tissue elements of the central nervous system (platinum method). *Scot. Med. Sci. J.,* **4**, 23.

Rubinstein, L. J. (1972). *Atlas of tumour pathology*, 2nd series, 6, *Tumours of the central nervous system.* (ed. Rubinstein, L. J.), American Armed Forces Institute of Pathology, Washington, DC.

Russell, D. S. & Rubinstein, L. J. (1977). *Pathology of tumours of the nervous system,* 4th edn. Edward Arnold, London.

Russell, W. R. & Whitty, C. W. M. (1952). Studies in traumatic epilepsy. I. Factors influencing the incidence of epilepsy after brain wounds. *J. Neurol. Neurosurg. Psychiat.,* **15**, 93–8.

Scholz, W. (1933). Über die Entstehung des Hirnbefundes bei der Epilepsie. *Z. ges. Neurol. Psychiat.*, **145**, 471.

Scoville, W. B. & Milner, B. (1957). Loss of recent memory after bilateral hippocampal lesions. *J. Neurol. Neurosurg. Psychiat.,* **20**, 11–21.

——, Dunsmore, R. H., Liberson, W. T., Henry, C. E. & Pepe, A. (1953). Observations on medial temporal lobotomy and uncotomy in the treatment of psychotic states: Preliminary review of 19 operative cases compared with 60 frontal lobectomy and undercutting cases. *Res. Pub. Assoc. Res. Nerv. Ment. Dis.,* **31**, 347–69.

Slater, E. & Beard, A. W. (1963). The schizophrenia-like psychoses of epilepsy. *Brit. J. Psychiat.,* **109**, 95–150.

Sommer, W. (1880). Erkrankung des Ammonshornes als aetiologisches Moment der Epilepsie. *Arch. Psychiat. NervKrankh.*, **10**, 631–75.

Spielmeyer, E. (1927). Die pathogenese des epileptischen Krampfes. *Z. ges. Neurol. Psychiat.*, **109**, 501–20 (1935).

Strich, S. J. (1976). Cerebral Trauma. In *Greenfield's Neuropathology*, 3rd edn., (eds. Blackwood, W. & Corsellis, J. A. N.), chap. 9, pp. 327–60. Edward Arnold, London.

Taylor, D. C. (1969(a)). Some psychiatric aspects of epilepsy. In *Current problems of neuropsychiatry, schizophrenia, epilepsy and the temporal lobe.* Brit. J. Psychiat. Spec. Pub. No. 4. (ed. Hetherington, R. N.), pp. 106–9.

—— (1969(b)). Differential rates of cerebral maturation between sexes and hemispheres. Evidence of epilepsy. *Lancet,* **2**, 140–2.

—— (1971). Ontogenesis of chronic epileptic psychoses: a reanalysis. *Psychol. Med.,* **1**, 247–53.

—— (1972). Mental state and temporal lobe epilepsy. A correlative account of patients treated surgically. *Epilepsia,* **13**, 727–65.

——(1975). Factors influencing the occurrence of schizophrenia-like psychosis in patients with temporal lobe epilepsy. *Psychol. Med.,* **5**, 249–54.

—— (1981(a)). Brain lesions, surgery, seizures and mental symptoms. In *Epilepsy and Psychiatry* (eds. Reynolds, E. H. & Trimble, M. R.). Churchill Livingstone, Edinburgh and London.

—— (1981(b)). The influences of sexual deviation on growth, development and disease. In *Scientific foundations of paediatrics,* 2nd edn., (eds. Davis, J. & Dobbin, J.). Heinemann, London.

—— & Falconer, M. A. (1968). Clinical socio-economic and psychological changes after temporal lobectomy for epilepsy. *Brit. J. Psychiat.,* **114**, 1247–61.

—— & Marsh, S. M. (1977). The strategy and implications of long term follow-up studies in epilepsy with a note on the cause of death. In *Epilepsy 8th International Symposium.* (ed. Penryck, J. K.). Raven Press, New York.

——, Falconer, M. A., Bruton, C. J. & Corsellis, J. A. N. (1971). Focal dysplasia of the cerebral cortex in epilepsy. *J. Neurol. Neurosurg. Psychiat.,* **34**, 369–87.

Trimble, M. R. (1981). The psychopathology of epilepsy. *Geigy Pharmaceuticals England,* 218–78.

Turner, J. (1907). The pathological anatomy and pathology of epilepsy. *J. Ment. Sci.* **53**, 1.

Turner, W. A. (1907). *Epilepsy: A study of the idiopathic disease.* Macmillan, New York.

Unterharnscheidt, F. & Higgins, L. S. (1969). Traumatic lesions of the brain and spinal cord due to nondeforming angular accelerations of the head. *Texas Reports Biol. Med.,* **27**, 127–66.

Urich, H. (1976). Malformation of the nervous system, perinatal damage and related conditions in early life. In *Greenfield's Neuropathology,* 3rd edn. (eds. Blackwood E. & Corsellis, J. A. N.), chap. 10, pp. 361–469. Edward Arnold, London.

Veith, G. (1970). Anatomische Studie über die Ammonshornsklerose im Epileptikergehirn. *Dt. Z. NervHeilk.,* **197**, 293–314.

Virchow, R. (1846). Ueber das granulirte Ansehen der Windungen der Gehirnventrikel. *Allg. Z. Psychiat.,* **3**, 424–50.

Vogt, C. & Vogt, O. (1922). Erkrankungen der Grosshirnrinde im Lichte der Topistik, Pathoklise und Pathoarchitektonik. *Psychol. Neurol. (Leipzig),* **28**, 1–171.

Weil, A. A. (1959). Ictal emotions occurring in temporal lobe dysfunction. *Arch. Neurol.* **1**, 101–11.

Wertham, F. & Wertham, Florence (1934). *The brain as an organ.* Macmillan, New York.

Williams, D. (1956). The structure of emotion reflected in epileptic experiences. *Brain,* **79**, 29–67.

Willis, R. A. (1947). *Pathology of tumours.* Butterworths, London.

World Health Organization (1979). International histological classification of tumours, No. 21. In *Histological typing of tumours of the central nervous system.* (ed. Zülch, K. J.), WHO., Geneva.

Zülch, K. J. (1956). Biologie und Pathologie der Hirngeschwülste. In *Handbuch der Neurochirurgie,* vol. 3. (eds. Olivecrona, H. & Tönnis, W.), Springer, Berlin.

Appendix I. List of patients in chronological order of operation from 1950–1975

Patient No.	Diagnostic group	Sex	Age at operation (yrs)	Age at first fit (yrs)	Side of lobec-tomy	Length of follow-up (yrs)
1	Indefinite	F	30	13	R	4
2	Trauma	M	25	Infancy	L	14
3	AHS	M	33	2	R	14
4	Double pathology	F	23	8/12	L	20
5	NAD	M	38	27	L	3
6	AHS	M	47	1/52	R	4
7	Alien tissue	M	11	7	L	2
8	AHS	M	14	8	L	2
9	NAD	F	25	21	L	12
10	Double pathology	M	15	5	R	2
11	NAD	F	39	35	L	10
12	NAD	F	28	15	R	9
13	NAD	F	27	9	R	3
14	Indefinite	F	33	17	L	20
15	Double pathology	F	21	7	L	2
16	Double pathology	F	32	5	R	10
17	Alien tissue	F	59	45	L	8
18	Developmental	F	30	4	L	6
19	NAD	M	29	24	L	1
20	AHS	F	16	2	R	8
21	NAD	F	25	5	R	No f/u
22	Trauma	M	48	29	R	7
23	Indefinite	M	14	9	L	3
24	AHS	M	17	11/12	L	18
25	AHS	F	20	8	L	7
26	Indefinite	M	28	13	R	No f/u
27	AHS	F	18	1	L	7
28	Double pathology	M	16	10	R	3

continued overleaf

Patient No.	Diagnostic group	Sex	Age at operation (yrs)	Age at first fit (yrs)	Side of lobec- tomy	Length of follow-up (yrs)
29	AHS	M	20	1	L	5
30	Alien tissue	M	38	28	L	12
31	AHS	M	22	1	L	No f/u
32	Alien tissue	M	19	13	R	2
33	NAD	M	54	36	L	11
34	AHS	F	23	3	L	5
35	AHS	F	30	17	L	12
36	AHS	F	27	16	R	20
37	AHS	M	37	2	L	11
38	NAD	M	49	39	L	17
39	NAD	F	16	7	L	1
40	NAD	M	21	13	R	9
41	AHS	M	42	3	L	4
42	Developmental	M	45	15	L	1
43	AHS	F	14	10/12	L	8
44	AHS	F	42	8/12	R	6
45	AHS	Ḿ	15	7	L	8
46	AHS	M	28	1	R	No f/u
47	NAD	F	39	28	L	2
48	Double pathology	M	25	2	R	17
49	Developmental	M	36	30	R	7
50	Indefinite	M	21	11	L	6
51	NAD	M	51	47	R	14
52	Indefinite	M	22	10	R	No f/u
53	AHS	M	19	9	L	3
54	Indefinite	M	27	3	L	14
55	Double pathology	M	27	18	R	15
56	AHS	M	14	2	L	2
57	Double pathology	M	27	3	L	5
58	Alien tissue	M	33	21	L	4
59	Developmental	M	32	18	R	10
60	Double pathology	M	9	3	R	13
61	AHS	M	19	3/12	L	12
62	Inflammatory	M	46	31	R	13
63	AHS	M	14	5	R	9
64	NAD	M	12	3	L	No f/u
65	Alien tissue	M	28	9	R	14
66	Alien tissue	M	20	4	L	2
67	Alien tissue	F	43	40	L	14

Patient No.	Diagnostic group	Sex	Age at operation (yrs)	Age at first fit (yrs)	Side of lobec- tomy	Length of follow-up (yrs)
68	AHS	M	12	8/12	R	5
69	Alien tissue	M	12	9	R	11
70	NAD	M	42	24	L	1
71	AHS	F	13	3	L	21
72	Alien tissue	F	35	34	R	8
73	AHS	F	24	6/12	R	1
74	AHS	F	13	9/12	L	1
75	AHS	M	23	1	L	3
76	Trauma	M	45	18	R	17
77	NAD	M	13	11	L	10
78	AHS	M	14	2	R	2
79	AHS	F	28	2	R	3
80	Indefinite	F	20	13	L	16
81	NAD	M	40	28	R	18
82	AHS	M	12	9/12	L	2
83	Inflammatory	M	36	12	R	10
84	AHS	F	13	10/12	R	13
85	AHS	M	22	11/12	R	6
86	Indefinite	M	31	4	L	1
87	AHS	M	23	12	L	18
88	AHS	M	33	30	L	9
89	AHS	F	17	8	L	18
90	AHS	M	13	10/12	L	3
91	Alien tissue	M	38	12	R	1
92	NAD	M	12	11	L	10
93	AHS	M	11	1	R	11
94	AHS	M	11	1	R	3
95	AHS	M	33	1	R	5
96	AHS	F	29	1	L	18
97	NAD	M	42	27	L	7
98	Double pathology	F	22	19	R	No f/u
99	Alien tissue	F	30	11	R	10
100	AHS	F	35	9	R	10
101	AHS	M	36	1	R	17
102	Alien tissue	F	17	Infancy	R	14
103	Alien tissue	F	51	41	R	15
104	Alien tissue	F	28	1	L	14
105	AHS	M	30	2	L	11
106	AHS	M	19	7	L	No f/u

Patient No.	Diagnostic group	Sex	Age at operation (yrs)	Age at first fit (yrs)	Side of lobectomy	Length of follow-up (yrs)
107	AHS	M	27	18/12	R	12
108	NAD	M	20	13	R	8
109	AHS	F	22	7	R	5
110	AHS	M	33	3	R	1
111	Indefinite	M	50	16	L	1
112	AHS	F	15	9	L	2
113	Trauma	F	19	12	L	16
114	AHS	M	36	3/12	L	19
115	AHS	M	25	18	R	1
116	AHS	M	54	29	L	2
117	Trauma	M	17	7	L	1
118	NAD	F	14	Birth	R	1
119	AHS	F	13	2/365	L	4
120	AHS	M	15	1	R	4
121	AHS	M	23	3	L	3
122	AHS	F	21	2	R	16
123	AHS	F	15	7/12	R	3
124	NAD	M	17	12	R	No f/u
125	Indefinite	M	38	30	L	10
126	NAD	M	22	1	R	7
127	NAD	M	24	5	R	12
128	AHS	M	44	2	L	No f/u
129	AHS	F	27	25	R	7
130	Inflammatory	M	10	5/12	L	3
131	Double pathology	F	36	35	R	10
132	Indefinite	F	18	5	R	7
133	Alien tissue	F	14	9	R	20
134	NAD	M	9	7	L	3
135	AHS	M	25	7/12	L	7
136	AHS	M	19	1	R	2
137	Double pathology	M	18	11	R	5
138	NAD	M	42	38	L	1
139	AHS	F	26	6	L	6
140	Indefinite	M	38	7	L	21
141	Alien tissue	M	46	32	L	15
142	Indefinite	M	25	7	L	15
143	AHS	M	20	1	R	4
144	Double pathology	M	16	4	L	14
145	AHS	M	18	2/365	L	10

Patient No.	Diagnostic group	Sex	Age at operation (yrs)	Age at first fit (yrs)	Side of lobec-tomy	Length of follow-up (yrs)
146	NAD	M	28	12	L	4
147	Double pathology	F	20	16	L	6
148	AHS	M	45	2	R	8
149	AHS	M	28	24	R	No f/u
150	Indefinite	F	42	4	R	No f/u
151	Indefinite	F	42	18	R	14
152	AHS	F	25	10/12	L	7
153	Alien tissue	M	32	18	L	10
154	AHS	M	29	6/12	R	18
155	Trauma	M	45	39	R	6
156	AHS	F	14	3	R	14
157	AHS	F	18	3	L	8
158	NAD	F	20	11	R	7
159	AHS	M	23	1	L	9
160	Alien tissue	M	32	13	L	3
161	AHS	M	25	1	L	4
162	Alien tissue	M	23	12	R	15
163	AHS	M	11	6/12	R	2
164	Double pathology	M	18	9	R	2
165	AHS	F	14	6	R	14
166	AHS	F	30	15	R	13
167	NAD	M	24	2	R	1
168	Alien tissue	M	35	23	R	19
169	Indefinite	M	16	2	R	8
170	AHS	F	20	2	L	No f/u
171	AHS	M	18	1	R	2
172	AHS	F	18	2	R	5
173	AHS	F	17	9	R	18
174	Alien tissue	F	18	6	L	17
175	AHS	M	16	4/12	L	6
176	AHS	M	35	26	L	2
177	NAD	F	17	7	R	4
178	Indefinite	F	28	1	R	16
179	NAD	M	25 } 27	19	R & L	2
180	Alien tissue	M	32	17	L	16
181	Alien tissue	M	19	16	R	12
182	Alien tissue	M	49	39	R	3
183	Alien tissue	F	19	14	R	13

Patient No.	Diagnostic group	Sex	Age at operation (yrs)	Age at first fit (yrs)	Side of lobec- tomy	Length of follow-up (yrs)
184	AHS	M	19	4	L	13
185	NAD	M	17	6	L	3
186	AHS	M	29	4	R	8
187	AHS	M	26	6/12	R	1
188	Alien tissue	F	14	7	L	3
189	AHS	M	29	1	R	5
190	AHS	F	20	7	R	No f/u
191	AHS	M	23	1	R	18
192	Indefinite	M	37	31	R	15
193	Inflammatory	F	28	4	L	12
194	Alien tissue	M	55	54	L	2
195	AHS	M	22	1	L	13
196	Indefinite	M	31	12	L	18
197	Alien tissue	M	11	8	R	1
198	AHS	F	17	1	R	12
199	Indefinite	M	47	30	R	17
200	NAD	F	22	16	R	12
201	Alien tissue	M	35	20	R	11
202	AHS	F	18	1	R	6
203	AHS	F	19	3/12	R	3
204	Indefinite	F	34	21	R	4
205	AHS	M	23	1/52	R	4
206	AHS	F	16	2	L	9
207	Double pathology	F	24	7	L	5
208	Alien tissue	F	2	1	L	22
209	Trauma	M	33	17	R	11
210	NAD	M	38	7	R	1
211	AHS	M	23	3	L	7
212	NAD	M	41	20	R	1
213	Alien tissue	M	17	12	L	6
214	Inflammatory	F	24	18	R	6
215	AHS	M	17	2	L	11
216	Alien tissue	M	19	6	R	18
217	Alien tissue	M	17	13	L	8
218	AHS	M	15	5	L	4
219	NAD	F	21	2	L	18
220	AHS	M	5	1	R	3
221	Indefinite	M	34	4	L	2
222	NAD	M	21	14	L	16

Patient No.	Diagnostic group	Sex	Age at operation (yrs)	Age at first fit (yrs)	Side of lobec-tomy	Length of follow-up (yrs)
223	AHS	M	44	29	L	6
224	Inflammatory	M	24	19	L	9
225	NAD	M	38	8	L	15
226	Alien tissue	M	16	2	L	4
227	Double pathology	F	17	2	R	20
228	AHS	F	22	1	L	20
229	AHS	M	38	8	R	11
230	Alien tissue	M	7	2	L	2
231	NAD	F	27	20	L	11
232	AHS	F	21	1	R	9
233	Indefinite	M	37	10	R	2
234	Alien tissue	F	15	8	L	1
235	Alien tissue	M	56	49	R	20
236	AHS	F	42	30	L	2
237	AHS	F	19	10/12	R	4
238	Alien tissue	M	20	5	R	2
239	AHS	M	22	7	L	3
240	Double pathology	M	22	5	L	12
241	AHS	M	17	3	R	2
242	Indefinite	M	39	32	R	2
243	AHS	F	19	9/12	L	11
244	AHS	F	28	1/12	L	12
245	AHS	F	30	4	R	15
246	Developmental	F	48	47	L	18
247	Inflammatory	M	9	5	L	5
248	NAD	F	45	7	L	20
249	Inflammatory	F	21	10	R	No f/u

f/u = follow-up
Age at first fit varied from birth to 55 years (mean age 10.60 yrs) (SD 11.74)
Age at operation varied between 2 months to 59 years (mean age 26.06 yrs) (SD 11.14)

Appendix II. Clinico-pathological results

GROUP 1. DEVELOPMENTAL LESIONS

Six patients (4 male and 2 female)

Clinical results

Case No.	Age at operation	Sex	Birth injury	Febrile convulsions	Pre-op. fit frequency
Diagnosis	Age at first fit	Side of lobectomy	Head injury	Status epilepticus	Other comments
18	30y	F	0	0	+ + +
Arachnoid cyst	4y	Left	0	0	AEG showed air-containing cyst at temporal pole
42	45y	M	0	0	+ +
White matter cyst	15y	Left	0	0	Schizophrenia
49	36y	M	0	0	+ + +
Epidermoid cyst	30y	Right	0	0	0
57*	27y	M	0	0	+ +
White matter cyst + Ammon's horn sclerosis	3y	Left	0	+	0
59	32y	M	0	0	Not known
Cortical malformation	18y	Right	+	0	Aggressive

Case No.	Age at operation	Sex	Birth injury	Febrile convulsions	Pre-op. fit frequency
Diagnosis	Age at first fit	Side of lobectomy	Head injury	Status epilepticus	Other comments
246 Cortical malformation	48y 47y	F Left	0 0	0 0	Not known 0

*Double pathology

Post-operative results

Case No.	Length of follow-up	Fit frequency	Personality and social adjustment	Comments
18	6y	Unaltered	Unaltered	
42	1y	Improved	Improved	
49	7y	Unaltered	Worse	Died – recurrence of patbology found at PM
57*	5y	Improved	Worse	Depressed, in psychiatric hospital
59	10y	Worse	Worse	Depressed, in psychiatric hospital
246	18y	Fit free	Normal life	Greatly improved

*Double pathology
Average length of follow-up 8 years.

Neuropathology

Case No.	Comments	Extent of resection
18	Thickened leptomeninges at uncus	Total
42	Cystic abnormality anterior to inferior horn of ventricle. Cyst wall of neuroglial tissue lined by ependyma	Total

Case No.	Comments	Extent of resection
49	Keratin-filled epidermoid cyst (1.5cm diameter) in parahippocampal and fusiform gyri	Total**
57*	Neuroglial cyst (similar to case 42) without an inner lining of ependyma	Total
59	Small heterotopic nodules in white matter below inferior horn of lateral ventricle	Total

*Double pathology   **Lesion recurred after 7 years.

GROUP 2.   TRAUMA

Ten patients (7 male and 3 female)
Clinical results

Case No.	Age at operation	Sex	Birth injury	Febrile convulsions	Pre-op. fit frequency
Diagnosis	Age at first fit	Side of lobectomy	Head injury	Status epilepticus	Other comments
2	25y	M	0	0	+ +
Subdural hygroma	Infancy	Left	+	0	0
4*	23y	F	+	0	+
Cortical scar + Ammon's horn sclerosis	8 mths	Left	+	+	0
22	48y	M	0	0	Not known
Cortical scar	29y	Right	+	0	0
55*	27y	M	0	0	+ +
Cortical scar + Ammon's horn sclerosis	18y	Right	+	0	0

Case No.	Age at operation	Sex	Birth injury	Febrile convulsions	Pre-op. fit frequency
Diagnosis	Age at first fit	Side of lobectomy	Head injury	Status epilepticus	Other comments
76	45y	M	0	0	+ + +
Cortical scar	18y	Right	+	0	0
113	19y	F	+	0	+ +
Cortical scar	12y	Left	+	0	Aggressive
117	17y	M	0	0	+ +
Cortical scar	7y	Left	+	0	0
155	45y	M	0	0	+ +
Cortical scar	39y	Right	0	0	0
209	33y	M	0	0	+ + +
White matter scar	17y	Right	+	0	Aggressive
227*	17y	F	+	+	+ + +
Cortical scar + Ammon's horn sclerosis	2y	Right	0	+	Aggressive

*Double Pathology

Post-operative results

Case No.	Length of follow-up	Fit frequency	Personality and social adjustment	Comments
2	14y	Unaltered	Unaltered	
4*	20y	Improved	Unaltered	Sometimes depressed
22	7y	Fit-free	Unaltered	
55*	15y	Fit-free	Normal life	Greatly improved. Running his own business

Case No.	Length of follow-up	Fit frequency	Personality and social adjustment	Comments
76	17y	Improved	Unaltered	Died – cause unrelated to epilepsy
113	16y	Unaltered	Worse	Difficult behaviour. In psychiatric care
117	1y	Worse	Unaltered	Died in epileptic fit
155	6y	Fit-free	Unaltered	
209	11y	Unaltered	Unaltered	
227*	20y	Fit-free	Normal life	Greatly improved

*Double pathology
Average length of follow-up: 13 years

Neuropathology

Case No.	Comments	Extent of resection
2	Subdural hygroma. Thickened and congested leptomeninges overlying temporal convexity	Total
4*	Focal cortical and white matter scar (uncus). Also AHS	Total
22	Focal cortical and white matter scar (in middle temporal gyrus (T2), inferior temporal gyrus (T3), fusiform and parahippocampal gyri)	Total
55*	Focal cortical and white matter scar (T3, T2, fusiform and parahippocampal gyri). Also AHS	Total
76	Focal cortical and white matter scar (Parahippocampal gyrus)	Total
113	Focal cortical and white matter scar (Very localized). (Parahippocampal gyrus)	Total
117	Focal cortical and white matter scar (Very localized). (T2)	Total
155	Focal cortical and white matter scar (T3, fusiform and uncus)	Total

Case No.	Comments	Extent of resection
209	Circumscribed focal abnormality in white matter (T3, T2). ? old burr hole site	Total
227*	Focal cortical and white matter scar (Diffuse damage). (T3 and T2). Also AHS	Total

*Double Pathology
T2 = middle temporal gyrus   T3 = inferior temporal gyrus

GROUP 3.   ALIEN TISSUE

3a. (i).   Astrocytic glial lesions
Nine patients (3 male and 6 female)

Clinical results

Case No.	Age at operation	Sex	Birth injury	Febrile convulsions	Pre-op. fit frequency
	Age at first fit	Side of lobectomy	Head injury	Status epilepticus	Other comments
17	59y	F	0	0	+ +
	45y	Left	0	0	0
67	43y	F	0	0	+ +
	40y	Left	0	0	Schizophrenic
72	35y	F	0	0	+ +
	34y	Right	0	0	0
147*	20y	F	0	0	+ + +
	16y	Left	0	0	0
183	19y	F	0	0	+ +
	14y	Right	0	0	0

Case No.	Age at operation	Sex	Birth injury	Febrile convulsions	Pre-op. fit frequency
	Age at first fit	Side of lo-bectomy	Head injury	Status epilepticus	Other comments
194	55y	M	0	0	+ +
	54y	Left	0	0	0
201	35y	M	0	0	+
	20y	Right	0	0	0
226	16y	M	0	0	+ +
	2y	Left	0	0	Aggressive
234	15y	F	0	0	+
	8y	Left	0	0	Aggressive

*Double pathology

Post-operative results

Case No.	Length of follow-up	Fit frequency	Personality and social adjustment	Comments
17	8y	Fit-free	Normal life	Greatly improved
67	14y	Fit-free	Normal life	Greatly improved
72	8y	Worse	Unaltered	Post-op. hemiparesis. Died – recurrence
147*	6y	Worse	Worse	Recurrent depression
183	13y	Fit-free	Normal life	Greatly improved
194	2y	Worse	Unaltered	Died – recurrence
201	11y	Improved	Normal life	
226	4y	Fit-free	Improved	
234	1y	Fit-free	Improved	'A changed person', cooperative, diligent, normal personality

*Double pathology   Average length of follow-up 7 years.

Neuropathology

Case No.	Predominant cell type	Cellular pleomorphism	Calcification	Abnormal vessel proliferation	Full removal suspected	Comments
		Mitoses	Cyst formation	Tissue necrosis		
17	Fibrillary astrocyte	+ + + 0	0 0	+ +	Yes	(Parahippocampal gyrus)
67	Protoplasmic astrocyte	+ 0	0 + + +	+ 0	Yes	(Parahippocampal and fusiform gyri)
72	Protoplasmic astrocyte	+ 0	0 + + +	+ 0	No	Lesion reached dorsal edge of resection (middle temporal gyrus (T2) and superior temporal gyrus (T1))
147*	Giant astrocyte	+ + + 0	0 0	+ + +	Yes	Anaplastic lesion (uncus, amygdaloid region and parahippocampal gyrus)
183	Protoplasmic astrocyte	0 0	0 + + +	0 0	Yes	Well-differentiated lesion (amygdaloid and parahippocampal gyrus)
194	Giant astrocyte	+ + + 0	0 0	+ +	No	Lesion reached edge of resection (difficult to assess extent of lesion)
201	Fibrillary astrocyte	+ 0	0 0	0 0	Yes	Well-differentiated lesion (uncus, amygdaloid and parahippocampal gyrus)

Case No.	Predom- inant cell type	Cellular pleomor- phism	Calcifica- tion	Abnormal vessel prolifera- tion	Full removal suspected	Comments
		Mitoses	Cyst formation	Tissue necrosis		
226	Proto- plasmic astrocyte	0 0	0 0	0 0	Yes	Very well differ- entiated lesion (amygdaloid)
234	Fibrillary astrocyte	0 0	0 0	0 0	Yes	Very well differ- entiated lesion (T3)

T1 = superior temporal gyrus   T2 = middle temporal gyrus   T3 = inferior temporal gyrus
*Double pathology

3a (ii).   *Oligodendrocytic glial lesions*
Six patients (4 male and 2 female)

Clinical results

Case No.	Age at operation	Sex	Birth injury	Febrile convulsions	Pre-op. fit frequency
	Age at first fit	Side of lobectomy	Head injury	Status epilepticus	Other comments
58	33y	M	0	0	+ + +
	21y	Left	0	0	0
103	51y	F	0	0	+
	41y	Right	0	0	0
131*	36y	F	0	0	Not known
	35y	Right	0	0	0
160	32y	M	0	0	+ +
	13y	Left	0	0	0

Case No.	Age at operation	Sex	Birth injury	Febrile convulsions	Pre-op. fit frequency
	Age at first fit	Side of lobectomy	Head injury	Status epilepticus	Other comments
216	19y	M	+	0	+ + +
	6y	Right	0	0	0
235	56y	M	0	0	+ +
	49y	Right	0	0	0

*Double pathology

Post-operative results

Case No.	Length of follow-up	Fit frequency	Personality and social adjustment	Comments
58	4y	Improved	Improved	Running his own business. Normal life
103	15y	Worse	Unaltered	Died – recurrence of lesion
131*	10y	Worse	Unaltered	Developing a dense left hemiparesis
160	3y	Improved	Improved	Now married. Learning to drive
216	18y	Greatly improved	Unaltered	Solitary. Unmarried. Inadequate
235	20y	Worse	Unaltered	Died – recurrence of lesion

*Double pathology
Average length of follow-up: 11 years

Neuropathology

Case No.	Cellular pleomorphism	Calcification	Abnormal vessel proliferation	Full removal suspected	Comments
	Mitoses	Cyst formation	Tissue necrosis		
58	0	0	0	Yes	Amygdaloid region
	0	0	0		
103	0	+	0	No	Lesion present at edge of resection (Uncus, amygdaloid, T1)
	0	+	0		
131*	+	0	0	No	Diffuse white matter spread. Also AHS
	0	0	0		
160	0	0	0	Yes	(Amygdaloid, hippo-campus and T1)
	0	+	0		
216	0	0	0	Yes	(Uncus, amygdaloid, hippocampus, parahip-pocampal, fusiform gyri)
	0	+	0		
235	0	0	0	No	Lesion present at edge of resection (Uncus, amygdaloid and T1)
	0	+	0		

*Double pathology   T1 = superior temporal gyrus

3a (iii).   *Mixed glial lesions*

Thirteen patients (9 male and 4 female)

Clinical results

Case No.	Age at operation	Sex	Birth injury	Febrile convulsions	Pre-op. fit frequency
	Age at first fit	Side of lobectomy	Head injury	Status epilepticus	Other comments
69	12y	M	0	0	+++
	9y	Right	0	0	0
91	38y	M	0	0	+++
	12y	Right	0	0	Schizophrenia
104	28y	F	0	0	+++
	1y	Left	0	0	0
133	14y	F	0	0	+++
	9y	Right	0	0	Aggressive
137*	18y	M	0	0	+++
	11y	Right	+	0	0
153	32y	M	0	0	+++
	18y	Left	0	0	0
164*	18y	M	0	0	++
	9y	Right	0	0	0
168	35y	M	0	0	+++
	23y	Right	0	0	0
181	19y	M	0	0	+++
	16y	Right	+	0	0
197	11y	M	0	0	+++
	8y	Right	0	0	0
207*	24y	F	0	0	++
	7y	Left	0	0	Aggressive
208	2y	F	0	0	+++
	1y	Left	0	0	Aggressive
240*	22y	M	0	0	+++
	5y	Left	0	0	0

*Double pathology

Post-operative results

Case No.	Length of follow-up	Fit frequency	Personality and social adjustment	Comments
69	11y	Improved	Normal life	Training as an accountant. Greatly improved
91	1y	Worse	Worse	Wildly schizophrenic. Died from natural causes after 1 yr
104	14y	Fit-free	Normal life	Greatly improved
133	20y	Fit-free	Normal life	Greatly improved
137*	5y	Fit-free	Normal life	Greatly improved
153	10y	Fit-free	Normal life	Greatly improved
164*	2y	Fit-free	Normal life	Improved
168	19y	Fit-free	Normal life	Greatly improved
181	12y	Fit-free	Normal life	Greatly improved
197	1y	Fit-free	Normal life	Improved
207*	5y	Fit-free	Normal life	Greatly improved
208	22y	Fit-free	Worse	Now schizophrenic
240*	12y	Fit-free	Normal life	Greatly improved

*Double pathology
Average length of follow-up: 10 years

Neuropathology

Case No.	Cellular pleomorphism	Calcification	Abnormal vessel proliferation	Full removal suspected	Comments
	Mitoses	Cyst formation	Tissue necrosis		
69	+	+++	+++	Yes	'Haemangioma Calcificans' (parahippocampal gyrus)
	0	+	0		

Case No.	Cellular pleomorphism	Calcification	Abnormal vessel proliferation	Full removal suspected	Comments
	Mitoses	Cyst formation	Tissue necrosis		
91	0	0	0	Yes	(Amygdaloid)
	0	0	0		
104	+	+++	0	Yes	(T3 and T2)
	0	0	0		
133	+	+++	0	Yes	(Amygdaloid and
	0	+	0		uncus)
137*	+	0	+	Yes	Large cyst adjacent
	0	+	0		to mixed glial lesion (Amygdaloid and uncus)
153	++	+	+++	Yes	'Haemangioma
	0	+	0		Calcificans' (parahippocampal gyrus and fusiform)
164*	0	+	+	Yes	Large cyst adjacent
	0	+	0		to mixed glial lesion (T3 and T2)
168	0	0	0	Yes	'Multicentric' lesion
	0	0	0		(Uncus, amygdaloid, hippocampus, fusiform and T3)
181	+	+++	+++	Yes	'Haemangioma
	0	+	0		Calcificans' (Amygdaloid, parahippocampal gyrus, T2 and T1)
197	+	+	0	Yes	(T3, T2 and T1)
	0	+	0		
207*	+	+	0	Yes	Amygdaloid, plus
	0	+	0		almost total AHS
208	0	+++	+	Yes	(Parahippocampal
	0	+	0		gyrus, fusiform, T3 and T2)

Case No.	Cellular pleomor- phism	Calcifica- tion	Abnormal vessel pro- liferation	Full removal suspected	Comments
	Mitoses	Cyst formation	Tissue necrosis		
240*	++ 0	0 0	0 0	Yes	Almost total AHS (Uncus, amygda- loid, hippocampus, parahippocampal gyrus)

*Double pathology
T1 = superior temporal gyrus   T2 = middle temporal gyrus   T3 = inferior temporal gyrus

3b.   *Neuronoglial lesions*

3b (i).   *Ganglioglial lesion*

Nine patients (6 male and 3 female)

Clinical results

Case No.	Age at operation	Sex	Birth injury	Febrile convulsions	Pre-op. fit frequency
	Age at first fit	Side of lobectomy	Head injury	Status epilepticus	Other comments
7	11y 7y	M Left	0 0	0 0	+++ 0
10*	15y 5y	M₁ Right	0 0	0 +	+ 0
60*	9y 3y	M Right	+ 0	0 0	+++ 0
98*	22y 19y	F Right	0 0	0 0	+++ 0
99	30y 11y	F Right	0 0	0 0	+ 0
102	17y Infancy	F Right	0 0	0 0	+ 0

Case No.	Age at operation	Sex	Birth injury	Febrile convulsions	Pre-op. fit frequency
	Age at first fit	Side of lobectomy	Head injury	Status epilepticus	Other comments
144*	16y	M	0	0	++
	4y	Left	0	0	0
162	23y	M	0	0	Not known
	12y	Right	0	0	0
230	7y	M	0	0	+++
	2y	Left	0	0	0

*Double pathology

Post-operative results

Case No.	Length of follow-up	Fit frequency	Personality and social adjustment	Comments
7	2y	Fit-free	Normal life	Improved
10*	2y	Fit-free	Worse	Aggressive and unmanageable
60*	13y	Improved	Worse	Became schizophrenic
98*	Not known	Not known	Not known	No follow-up
99	10y	Fit-free	Worse	Has become schizophrenic
102	14y	Fit-free	Worse	Has become schizophrenic
144*	14y	Fit-free	Worse	Became schizophrenic. Committed suicide
162	15y	Fit-free	Normal	Died – unrelated cause
230	2y	Worse	Worse	Aggressive. Behaviour problem

*Double pathology
Average length of follow-up 9 years.

Neuropathology

Case No.	Cellular pleomor- phism	Calcifica- tion	Abnormal vessel pro- liferation	Full removal suspected	Comments
	Mitoses	Cyst for- mation	Tissue necrosis		
7	+	+++	0	Yes	(Parahippocampal
	0	0	0		gyrus)
10*	+	+	0	Yes	(Uncus and amyg-
	0	0	0		daloid). Also AHS
60*	+	0	0	Yes	(Uncus, amygdaloid
	0	0	0		and parahippocam-
					pal gyrus). Also
					AHS
98*	++	0	0	Yes	Ependymal-lined
	0	+	0		development cyst
					present (Parahippo-
					campal gyrus, fusi-
					form, T3 and T2)
99	++	0	+	Yes	(Amygdaloid, para-
	0	+	0		hippocampal gyrus,
					hippocampus)
102	+	++	0	Yes	(Uncus, amygda-
	0	0	0		loid, hippocampus
					and parahippo-
					campal gyrus)
144*	+	+	+	Yes	(Uncus and amyg-
	0	+	0		daloid). Also AHS
162	+	++	+	Yes	(Uncus and para-
	0	+	0		hippocampal gyrus)
230	+	+	+	Yes	(Uncus, amygda-
	0	0	0		loid, hippocampus,
					parahippocampal
					and fusiform gyri)

*Double pathology
T2 = middle temporal gyrus   T3 = inferior temporal gyrus

3b (ii). *Cortical dysplasia*

Eight patients (7 male and 1 female)

Clinical results

Case No.	Age at operation	Sex	Birth injury	Febrile convulsions	Pre-op. fit frequency
	Age at first fit	Side of lobectomy	Head injury	Status epilepticus	Other comments
65	28y	M	0	0	++
	3y	Right	+	0	0
66	20y	M	0	0	+++
	4y	Left	0	0	Aggressive
141	46y	M	0	0	++
	31y	Left	+	0	0
174	18y	F	+	0	++
	6y	Left	0	0	Aggressive
182	49y	M	0	0	+++
	39y	Right	0	0	0
213	17y	M	0	0	+
	12y	Left	0	0	Aggressive
217	17y	M	0	0	++
	13y	Left	0	0	Aggressive
238	20y	M	0	0	++
	5y	Right	0	0	0

Post-operative results

Case No.	Length of follow-up	Fit frequency	Personality and social adjustment	Comments
65	14y	Fit-free	Normal life	Greatly improved
66	2y	Fit-free	Normal life	
141	15y	Improved	Improved	Died (unrelated cause)

Case No.	Length of follow-up	Fit frequency	Personality and social adjustment	Comments
174	17y	Unaltered	Unaltered	
182	3y	Improved	Improved	
213	6y	Improved	Unaltered	
217	8y	Unaltered	Unaltered	Very aggressive – in custodial care
238	2y	Fit-free	Improved	Post-operative hemiparesis

Average length of follow-up 8 years.

Neuropathology

Case No.	Cellular pleomor-phism	Calcifica-tion	Abnormal vessel pro-liferation	Full removal suspected	Comments
	Mitoses	Cyst for-mation	Tissue necrosis		
65	+ 0	0 0	0 0	Yes	(Fusiform, T3, T2)
66	+ 0	0 0	0 0	Yes	(Amygdaloid, T2, T1)
141	+	0	0	Yes	(Fusiform and T3)
174	+ 0	0 0	0 0	Yes	Hippocampus
182	+ 0	0 0	0 0	Yes	T2 and T1
213	+ 0	0 0	0 0	Yes	T1
217	+ 0	0 0	0 0	Yes	(Parahippocampal gyrus, fusiform, T3, T2, T1)
238	+ 0	0 0	0 0	Yes	T1

T1 = superior temporal gyrus   T2 = middle temporal gyrus   T3 = inferior temporal gyrus

3c. *Vascular abnormalities*

Four patients (3 male and 1 female)

Clinical results

Case No.	Age at operation	Sex	Birth injury	Febrile convulsions	Pre-op. fit frequency
	Age at first fit	Side of lobectomy	Head injury	Status epilepticus	Other comments
28*	16y	M	0	0	++
	10y	Right	0	0	Aggressive
30	38y	M	0	0	+++
	28y	Left	0	0	Aggressive, paranoid
32	19y	M	0	0	+++
	13y	Right	0	0	0
188	14y	F	0	0	+
	7y	Left	0	0	Aggressive

*Double pathology

Post-operative results

Case No.	Length of follow-up	Fit frequency	Personality and social adjustment	Comments
28*	3y	Unaltered	Unaltered	
30	12y	Improved	Unaltered	Post-operative dysphasia
32	2y	Fit-free	Worse	Died – suicide
188	3y	Improved	Improved	

*Double pathology
Average length of follow-up 5 years.

Neuropathology

Case No.	Cellular pleomor- phism	Calcifica- tion	Abnormal vessel pro- liferation	Full removal suspected	Comments
	Mitoses	Cyst formation	Tissue necrosis		
28*	0	0	+	Yes	Classical AHS.
	0	0	0		Arterio-venous malformation (T2)
30	0	+	+	Yes	Cavernous angioma
	0	0	0		(parahippocampal gyrus)
32	0	+	+	Yes	Cavernous angioma
	0	0	0		(fusiform T3 and T2)
188	0	+	+	Yes	Cavernous angioma
	0	0	0		(T1)

*Double pathology
T1 = superior temporal gyrus   T2 = middle temporal gyrus
T3 = inferior temporal gyrus

GROUP 4. AMMON'S HORN SCLEROSIS

4a.   Ammon's horn sclerosis: single lesion

107 patients (63 male and 44 female)

Clinical results

Case No.	Age at operation	Sex	Birth injury	Febrile convulsions	Pre-op. fit frequency
	Age at first fit	Side of lobectomy	Head injury	Status epilepticus	Other comments
3	33y	M	0	0	++
	2y	Right	+	+	0
6	47y	F	NK	NK	+++
	1wk	Right	0	0	0

Case No.	Age at operation	Sex	Birth injury	Febrile convulsions	Pre-op. fit frequency
	Age at first fit	Side of lobectomy	Head injury	Status epilepticus	Other comments
8	14y	M	0	0	+++
	8y	Left	+	0	0
20	16y	F	0	+	+++
	2y	Right	0	0	0
24	17y	M	0	+	++
	1y	Left	0	+	0
25	20y	F	0	0	+
	8y	Left	0	0	Malaria aged 1y. Schizophrenic
27	18y	F	0	+	++
	1y	Left	0	0	0
29	20y	M	+	0	++
	1y	Left	0	0	0
31	22y	M	0	+	+++
	1y	Left	0	0	0
34	23y	F	0	+	+++
	3y	Left	0	+	0
35	30y	F	0	NK	++
	17y	Left	0	0	Whooping cough at 6 months
36	27y	F	0	0	0
	16y	Right	0	0	Whooping cough at 2 years
37	37y	M	+	0	++
	2y	Left	0	+	0
41	42y	M	0	+	+++
	3y	Left	0	0	0
43	14y	F	0	0	+
	1y	Left	0	+	Strong F.H. of epilepsy

Case No.	Age at operation	Sex	Birth injury	Febrile convulsions	Pre-op. fit frequency
	Age at first fit	Side of lobectomy	Head injury	Status epilepticus	Other comments
44	32y	F	0	+	++
	1y	Right	0	0	0
45	15y	M	+	0	+
	7y	Left	+	0	Aggressive
46	28y	M	0	+	+++
	1y	Right	0	0	Aggressive
53	19y	M	0	0	+++
	9y	Left	0	0	Aggressive
56	14y	M	0	0	+
	2y	Left	0	0	Meningitis at 1y
61	19y	M	+	+	+
	3 mths	Left	0	0	Schizophrenic
63	14y	M	+	0	+++
	5y	Right	0	0	Aggressive
68	12y	M	0	+	+
	1y	Right	0	+	Aggressive
71	13y	F	0	+	+
	3y	Left	0	0	Measles, encephalitis, and hemiplegia
73	24y	F	0	+	+++
	6 mths	Right	0	0	0
74	13y	F	0	+	+++
	1y	Left	0	0	0
75	23y	M	0	+	++
	1y	Left	0	+	Aggressive
78	14y	M	0	+	++
	2y	Right	0	0	Aggressive
79	28y	F	0	0	++
	2y	Left	0	0	0
82	12y	M	0	+	++
	1y	Left	0	0	Aggressive

Case No.	Age at operation	Sex	Birth injury	Febrile convulsions	Pre-op. fit frequency
	Age at first fit	Side of lobectomy	Head injury	Status epilepticus	Other comments
84	13y	F	0	0	+++
	1y	Right	0	0	0
85	22y	M	0	+	++
	1y	Right	0	0	0
87	23y	M	+	0	++
	12y	Left	0	0	0
88	33y	M	0	0	++
	30y	Left	+	0	0
89	17y	F	0	0	++
	8y	Left	0	0	0
90	13y	M	0	+	++
	1y	Right	0	+	Aggressive
93	11y	M	0	0	+++
	1y	Right	0	0	Aggressive
94	11y	M	0	+	+++
	1y	Right	0	+	0
95	33y	M	0	0	+++
	1y	Right	+	+	0
96	29y	F	0	+	+++
	1y	Left	0	+	Measles, encephalitis. Schizophrenic
100	35y	F	0	0	++
	9y	Right	0	+	Meningitis 3y
101	36y	M	0	+	+
	1y	Right	0	0	Mastoid op.
105	30y	M	+	0	++
	2y	Left	0	0	Schizophrenic
106	19y	M	0	0	+++
	2y	Left	0	0	Aggressive
107	27y	M	+	+	++
	1y	Right	+	0	0

Case No.	Age at operation / Age at first fit	Sex / Side of lobectomy	Birth injury / Head injury	Febrile convulsions / Status epilepticus	Pre-op. fit frequency / Other comments
109	22y	F	+	+	+++
	7y	Right	0	+	0
110	33y	M	0	+	++
	3y	Right	0	0	Schizophrenic
112	15y	F	0	0	++
	9y	Left	0	0	0
114	36y	M	0	+	+++
	3 mths	Left	0	0	0
115	25y	M	0	0	++
	18y	Right	+	0	0
116	54y	M	0	0	+
	29y	Left	+	0	Severe electric shock
119	13y	F	0	+	++
	2 days	Left	0	0	Aggressive
120	15y	M	0	+	++
	1y	Right	0	0	0
121	23y	M	0	0	+++
	3y	Left	0	0	0
122	21y	F	+	0	++
	2y	Right	0	0	0
123	15y	F	+	+	Not known
	1y	Right	0	0	0
128	44y	M	0	0	++
	2y	Left	0	0	Aggressive
129	27y	F	0	0	++
	25y	Right	0	0	Mastoid operation
135	25y	M	0	+	++
	1y	Left	0	0	0
136	19y	M	0	+	++
	1y	Right	0	0	0
139	26y	F	+	0	++
	6y	Left	0	0	0

Case No.	Age at operation	Sex	Birth injury	Febrile convulsions	Pre-op. fit frequency
	Age at first fit	Side of lobectomy	Head injury	Status epilepticus	Other comments
143	20y	M	0	+	++
	1y	Right	0	+	Aggressive
145	18y	M	0	0	+
	3 days	Left	0	0	0
148	45y	M	0	0	+++
	2y	Right	+	0	Schizophrenic
149	28y	M	0	0	Not known
	24y	Right	0	0	Aggressive. Mastoid operation
152	25y	F	+	+	++
	1y	Left	0	0	Aggressive
154	29y	M	0	+	+++
	6 mths	Right	0	0	0
156	14y	F	0	+	+++
	3y	Right	0	0	0
157	18y	F	0	+	++
	3y	Left	0	+	Rubella, encephalitis
159	23y	M	+	0	+
	1y	Left	0	0	Aggressive
161	25y	M	0	+	+++
	1y	Left	0	+	0
163	11y	M	0	+	+++
	6 mths	Right	0	0	0
165	14y	F	0	+	+++
	6y	Right	0	+	Aggressive
166	30y	F	0	0	++
	15y	Right	0	0	0
170	20y	F	0	+	++
	2y	Left	0	0	0
171	18y	M	0	+	++
	1y	Right	0	0	0

Case No.	Age at operation	Sex	Birth injury	Febrile convulsions	Pre-op. fit frequency
	Age at first fit	Side of lobectomy	Head injury	Status epilepticus	Other comments
172	18y	F	0	0	+
	2y	Right	0	0	0
173	18y	F	0	0	+++
	9y	Right	0	0	0
175	16y	M	+	0	+
	4 mths	Left	0	0	0
176	35y	M	0	0	+++
	26y	Left	0	0	0
184	19y	M	+	+	++
	4y	Left	0	0	0
186	29y	M	0	0	++
	4y	Right	0	0	0
187	26y	M	0	0	+
	6 mths	Right	0	0	0
189	29y	M	0	+	+
	1y	Right	0	0	0
190	20y	F	+	0	+++
	7y	Right	0	0	0
191	23y	M	0	+	+++
	1y	Right	0	0	0
195	22y	M	0	+	++
	1y	Left	0	0	Schizophrenic. Aggressive
198	17y	F	0	0	++
	1y	Right	0	0	0
202	18y	F	0	0	+
	1y	Right	+	+	0
203	19y	F	+	0	++
	3 mths	Right	0	0	Aggressive/MD
205	23y	M	0	0	++
	1 wk	Right	0	0	Strong FH of epilepsy
206	16y	F	+	0	+++
	2y	Left	0	0	Aggressive

| Case No. | Age at operation | Sex | Birth injury | Febrile convulsions | Pre-op. fit frequency |
	Age at first fit	Side of lobectomy	Head injury	Status epilepticus	Other comments
211	23y	M	0	+	++
	3y	Left	0	0	Aggressive
215	17y	M	0	0	+++
	2y	Left	0	+	Aggressive/poliomyelitis
218	15y	M	0	0	+++
	5y	Left	0	0	0
220	5y	M	0	+	+++
	1y	Right	0	0	0
223	44y	M	0	0	++
	29y	Left	0	0	Aggressive/ mastoid operation
228	22y	F	0	+	+
	1y	Left	0	0	Schizophrenic
229	38y	M	0	0	++
	28y	Right	+	0	0
232	21y	F	0	+	++
	1y	Right	0	0	0
236	42y	F	0	0	+++
	30y	Left	0	0	Toxaemia of pregnancy
237	19y	F	0	0	+
	1y	Right	0	0	0
239	22y	M	0	+	+++
	7y	Left	0	+	Aggressive
241	17y	M	0	0	+
	9y	Right	0	0	Meningitis/aggressive
243	19y	F	+	0	++
	1y	Left	0	0	0
244	28y	F	0	+	++
	1 mth	Left	0	0	0
245	30y	F	0	0	+
	4y	Right	0	0	0

NK = not known   MD = mental deficiency   FH = family history

Post-operative results
Follow-up information was available in 100 of the 107 cases

Case No.	Length of follow-up	Fit frequency	Personality and social adjustment	Comments
3	14y	Fit-free	Normal life	Greatly improved
6	4y	Improved	Normal life	
8	2y	Fit-free	Normal life	
20	8y	Fit-free	Normal life	Greatly improved
24	18y	Worse	Worse	Very aggressive
25	7y	Fit-free	Normal life	Greatly improved
27	7y	Fit-free	Unaltered	
29	5y	Unaltered	Unaltered	Died after a fit (drowned)
34	5y	Fit-free	Normal life	Greatly improved
35	12y	Fit-free	Normal life	Greatly improved
36	20y	Fit-free	Normal life	Greatly improved
37	11y	Fit-free	Normal life	Greatly improved
41	4y	Improved	Normal life	
43	8y	Improved	Normal life	
44	6y	Fit-free	Normal life	Greatly improved
45	8y	Worse	Worse	Aggressive. Sexually deviant. In top security prison hospital
53	3y	Fit-free	Improved	
56	2y	Fit-free	Improved	
61	12y	Fit-free	Normal life	Greatly improved
63	9y	Unaltered	Unaltered	Aggressive
68	5y	Improved	Unaltered	Aggressive
71	21y	Fit-free	Unaltered	Post-operative hemiparesis
73	1y	Fit-free	Improved	
74	1y	Fit-free	Improved	
75	3y	Fit-free	Improved	
78	2y	Improved	Improved	
79	3y	Fit-free	Normal life	

Case No.	Length of follow-up	Fit frequency	Personality and social adjustment	Comments
82	2y	Fit-free	Unaltered	Aggressive
84	13y	Fit-free	Normal life	Greatly improved
85	6y	Fit-free	Normal life	Greatly improved
87	18y	Fit-free	Normal life	Greatly improved
88	9y	Improved	Worse	Depressed (in psychiatric hospital)
89	18y	Fit-free	Normal life	Greatly improved
90	3y	Fit-free	Normal life	
93	11y	Fit-free	Unaltered	Aggressive. In prison
94	3y	Fit-free	Normal life	
95	5y	Fit-free	Normal life	Greatly improved
96	18y	Fit-free	Worse	Schizophrenic
100	10y	Improved	Normal life	
101	17y	Unaltered	Unaltered	Impotent
105	11y	Fit-free	Normal life	Greatly improved
107	12y	Fit-free	Unaltered	Impotent
109	5y	Improved	Normal life	
110	1y	Worse	Unaltered	Became schizophrenic. Died in status epilepticus
112	2y	Fit-free	Normal life	
114	19y	Fit-free	Normal life	Greatly improved
115	1y	Unaltered	Unaltered	
116	2y	Improved	Improved	
119	4y	Fit-free	Worse	Schizophrenic. Aggressive
120	4y	Fit-free	Normal life	
121	3y	Improved	Normal life	
122	16y	Fit-free	Normal life	Greatly improved
123	3y	Fit-free	Normal life	
129	7y	Worse	Worse	Depressed – suicidal
135	7y	Fit-free	Normal life	Greatly improved

Case No.	Length of follow-up	Fit frequency	Personality and social adjustment	Comments
136	2y	Fit-free	Normal life	Improved
139	6y	Worse	Worse	Depressed. Died – suicide
143	4y	Unaltered	Unaltered	Aggressive. Died after a fit (drowned)
145	10y	Unaltered	Unaltered	
148	8y	Improved	Unaltered	Paranoid schizophrenic
152	7y	Improved	Worse	Depressed and aggressive
154	18y	Fit-free	Normal life	Greatly improved
156	14y	Improved	Normal life	
157	8y	Unaltered	Unaltered	Depressed
159	9y	Fit-free	Normal life	Greatly improved
161	4y	Improved	Normal life	
163	2y	Fit-free	Normal life	
165	14y	Fit-free	Unaltered	Aggressive
166	13y	Unaltered	Unaltered	
171	2y	Fit-free	Normal life	
172	5y	Fit-free	Normal life	Greatly improved
173	18y	Fit-free	Normal life	Greatly improved
175	6y	Improved	Unaltered	Aggressive
176	2y	Worse	Unaltered	Post-op. hemiplegia. Died – cause unknown
184	13y	Fit-free	Normal life	Greatly improved
186	8y	Fit-free	Normal life	Greatly improved
187	1y	Fit-free	Normal life	
189	5y	Unaltered	Unaltered	
191	18y	Improved	Normal life	
195	13y	Unaltered	Unaltered	Aggressive and schizophrenic
198	12y	Fit-free	Normal life	Greatly improved

Case No.	Length of follow-up	Fit frequency	Personality and social adjustment	Comments
202	6y	Fit-free	Improved	
203	3y	Unaltered	Unaltered	Aggressive
205	4y	Fit-free	Normal life	
206	9y	Worse	Worse	Aggressive and depressed. Died – suicide
211	7y	Fit-free	Normal life	Greatly improved
215	11y	Unaltered	Unaltered	Aggressive
218	4y	Fit-free	Normal life	At university
220	3y	Fit-free	Normal life	
223	6y	Fit-free	Worse	Schizophrenic
228	20y	Improved	Unaltered	Schizophrenic
229	11y	Unaltered	Unaltered	
232	9y	Fit-free	Unaltered	Depressed
236	2y	Improved	Improved	
237	4y	Fit-free	Improved	Gold medal ballroom dancer
239	3y	Improved	Improved	
241	2y	Fit-free	Improved	
243	11y	Fit-free	Normal life	Greatly improved
244	12y	Fit-free	Normal life	Greatly improved
245	15y	Fit-free	Normal life	Greatly improved

Average length of follow-up: 8 years. Number of cases: 100
Effect of operation on fit pattern:
 Greatly improved (37), Improved (43), Unaltered (13), Worse (7).
Effect of operation on personality and social adjustment:
 Greatly improved (34), Improved (30), Unaltered (26), Worse (10).

Neuropathology

Case No.	Type of Ammon's horn sclerosis	White matter gliosis	Amygdaloid damage	Nerve cell loss in adjacent cerebral cortex
3	Classical	++	0	0
6	Total	+	+	0
8	Total	++	+	0
20	Total	+	+	0
24	Classical	++	+	0
25	Classical	++	+++	0
27	Classical	++	+	0
29	Total	+	++	0
31	Total	+++	++	0
34	Total	+	++	0
35	Classical	+	0	0
36	Classical	+	0	0
37	Total	+	++	0
41	Classical	++	+	0
43	Total	++	+	0
44	Classical	+	+	0
45	End folium	+	0	+
46	Total	++	++	+
53	Total	++	++	++
56	Classical	++	NPA	0
61	Total	++	++	+
63	Classical	+	+	0
68	Classical	+	+	0
71	Total	++	NPA	++
73	Total	++	++	+
74	Total	++	++	0
75	Classical	+	+	0
78	Classical	++	++	0
79	Classical	+	+	0
82	Classical	+	+	0
84	Classical	+	+	0

Case No.	Type of Ammon's horn sclerosis	White matter gliosis	Amygdaloid damage	Nerve cell loss in adjacent cerebral cortex
85	Classical	+	0	0
87	End folium	++	+	0
88	Total	++	+	+
89	Classical	+	+	0
90	Total	++	++	+
93	Total	++	++	0
94	Classical	+	++	0
95	Total	+++	++	+
96	Classical	+	+	0
100	Classical	+++	++	0
101	Total	++	++	0
105	Classical	++	++	0
106	Classical	+	NPA	0
107	Classical	+	+	0
109	Classical	++	++	0
110	Total	+ +	+	0
112	Classical	++	+	0
114	Classical	+	+	0
115	Classical	+	+	+
116	Total	++	+	+
119	Classical	+++	+++	+
120	Classical	++	NPA	0
121	Total	++	++	+
122	Classical	+	0	0
123	Total	++	+	+
128	Classical	+	+	0
129	Classical	+	0	0
135	Classical	+	NPA	0
136	Total	+	+	0
139	Classical	+	+	0
143	Total	++	++	0
145	Classical	+++	++	+

Case No.	Type of Ammon's horn sclerosis	White matter gliosis	Amygdaloid damage	Nerve cell loss in adjacent cerebral cortex
148	Total	++	++	0
149	Classical	+++	+	0
152	Classical	+	+	0
154	Classical	+	++	+
156	Classical	+	+	0
157	Total	+	+	0
159	Classical	+	+	0
161	Total	+ +	+ +	0
163	Total	+++	+	+
165	Classical	++	0	0
166	Classical	++	0	0
170	Total	++	+	0
171	Total	++	NPA	0
172	Classical	++	+	0
173	Classical	+	NPA	0
175	Classical	+	NPA	0
176	End folium	++	NPA	0
184	Classical	++	+	0
186	Total	+++	++	+
187	Classical	+	+	0
189	Total	++	NPA	0
190	Total	++	+	+
191	Classical	++	NPA	0
195	Classical	+	0	0
198	Classical	++	+	0
202	Classical	+	+	0
203	Classical	+++	++	++
205	Classical	+++	++	0
206	Classical	+	+	0
211	Total	++	NPA	0
215	Total	+	+	0
218	Total	++	+	+

Case No.	Type of Ammon's horn sclerosis	White matter gliosis	Amygdaloid damage	Nerve cell loss in adjacent cerebral cortex
220	Total	++	++	+
223	End folium	++	0	0
228	Total	++	NPA	++
229	Classical	+	+	0
232	Total	++	+	+
236	Total	++	+	0
237	Classical	++	+	+
239	Total	++	++	+
241	Classical	+	NPA	0
243	Classical	+	+	+
244	Classical	++	NPA	0
245	Classical	+	+	0

NPA = not possible to assess
Total number of patients with AHS: 107
Number of patients with classical AHS: 61 (57%)
Number of patients with total AHS: 42 (39%)
Number of patients with end folium sclerosis: 4 (4%)

Ammon's horn sclerosis: Double pathology group
15 patients (8 male, 7 female)
Clinical results

Case No.	Age at operation	Sex	Birth injury	Febrile convulsions	Pre-op. fit frequency
	Age at first fit	Side of lobectomy	Head injury	Status epilepticus	Other comments
4	23y	F	+	0	+
	8 mths	Left	+	+	0
10	15y	M	0	0	+
	5y	Right	0	+	0
15	21y	F	0	0	+
	7y	Left	0	0	0
16	32y	F	0	0	+++
	6y	Right	0	0	0
28	16y	M	0	0	++
	10y	Right	0	0	Aggressive
48	25y	M	0	0	+++
	2y	Right	0	0	0
55	27y	M	0	0	++
	18y	Right	+	0	0
57	27y	M	0	+	++
60	9y	M	+	0	++
	3y	Right	0	0	0
131	36y	F	0	0	Not known
	35y	Right	0	0	0
144	16y	M	0	0	++
	4y	Left	0	0	0
147	20y	F	0	0	+++
	16y	Left	0	0	0
207	24y	F	0	0	++
	7y	Left	0	0	Aggressive
227	17y	F	+	0	Not known
	2y	Right	0	+	0
240	22y	M	0	0	+++
	5y	Left	0	0	0

Post-operative results

Case No.	Length of follow-up	Fit frequency	Personality and social adjustment	Comments
4	20y	Improved	Unaltered	Recurrent depression
10	2y	Fit-free	Worse	Aggressive and unmanageable
15	2y	Fit-free	Normal life	
16	10y	Fit free	Unaltered	Post-op. hemiplegia
28	3y	Unaltered	Unaltered	Still aggressive
48	17y	Fit-free	Unaltered	Athetotic movements
55	15y	Fit-free	Normal life	Greatly improved
57	5y	Improved	Worse	Depressed, in psychiatric hospital
60	13y	Improved	Worse	Became schizophrenic
131	10y	Worse	Unaltered	Developing a dense hemiparesis
144	14y	Fit-free	Worse	Became schizophrenic, committed suicide
147	6y	Worse	Worse	Recurrent depression
207	5y	Fit-free	Normal life	Greatly improved
227	20y	Fit-free	Normal life	Greatly improved
240	12y	Fit-free	Normal life	Greatly improved

Average length of follow-up: 10 years. Number of cases: 15
Effect of operation on fit pattern:
  Greatly improved (7), Improved (5), Unaltered (1), Worse (2).
Effect of operation on personality and social adjustment:
  Greatly improved (4), Improved (1), Unaltered (5), Worse (5)

Neuropathology

Case No.	Type of Ammon's horn sclerosis	Other pathology	Extent of resection
57	Total	Developmental lesion (cyst)	Complete
4	Classical	Trauma (cortical scar)	Complete
55	Classical	Trauma (cortical scar)	Complete
227	Total	Trauma (cortical scar)	Complete
10	Total	Alien tissue (neuronoglial lesion)	Complete
28	Classical	Alien tissue (vascular lesion)	Complete
60	Total	Alien tissue (neuronoglial lesion)	Complete
131	Classical	Alien tissue (oligodendrocytic lesion)	Complete
144	Total	Alien tissue (neuronoglial lesion)	Complete
147	Total	Alien tissue (astrocytic lesion)	Complete
207	Total	Alien tissue (mixed glial lesion)	Complete
240	Total	Alien tissue (mixed glial lesion)	Complete
15	Classical	Inflammatory lesion	Incomplete
16	Classical	Inflammatory lesion	Complete
48	Total	Inflammatory lesion	Incomplete

Total number of patients with AHS: 15
Number of patients with classical AHS: 6 (40%)
Number of patients with total AHS: 9 (60%)

GROUP 5. INFLAMMATORY

Eleven patients (6 male and 5 female)

Clinical results

Case No.	Age at operation	Sex	Birth injury	Febrile convulsions	Pre-op. fit frequency
Neuropathological diagnosis	Age at first fit	Side of lobectomy	Head injury	Status epilepticus	Other
15	21y	F	0	0	+++
Meningitis/AHS*	7y	Left	0	0	Meningitis
16	32y	F	0	0	+++
Abscess/AHS*	5y	Right	0	0	Cerebral abscess
48	25y	M	0	0	+++
Meningitis/AHS*	2y	Right	0	0	Meningitis
62	46y	M	0	0	++
Abscess	5y	Right	+	0	Cerebral abscess
83	36y	M	0	0	++
Abscess	12y	Right	0	0	Cerebral abscess
130	10y	M	0	0	Not known
Encephalitis	6mths	Left	0	0	Aggressive/ encephalitis
193	28y	F	0	+	+++
Meningitis	4y	Left	0	0	Meningitis
214	24y	F	0	0	Not known
Meningitis	18y	Right	0	0	0
224	24y	M	0	0	++
Abscess	19y	Left	0	0	Cerebral abscess
247	24y	M	0	0	+++
Encephalitis	5y	Left	+	0	Aggressive
249	21y	F	0	0	Not known
Meningitis	10y	Right	0	0	Meningitis

*Double pathology

Post-operative results

Case No.	Length of follow-up	Fit frequency	Personality and social adjustment	Comments
15*	2y	Fit-free	Normal life	
16*	10y	Fit-free	Unaltered	(Post-op. hemiplegia)
48*	17y	Fit-free	Unaltered	Bizarre athetoid movements
62	13y	Improved	Unaltered	
83	10y	Improved	Improved	
130	3y	Improved	Worse	Died in a fit
193	12y	Unaltered	Unaltered	
214	6y	Improved	Improved	
224	9y	Improved	Improved	
247	5y	Unaltered	Unaltered	In an epileptic colony. Dysphasic
249	—	—	—	No follow-up

*Double pathology
Follow-up information was available in 10 cases
Average length of follow-up: 8.7 years
Effect of operation on fit pattern:
    Greatly improved (2), Improved (6), Unaltered (2), Worse (0)
Effect of operation on personality and social adjustment:
    Greatly improved (0), Improved (4), Unaltered (5), Worse (1)

Neuropathology

Case No.	Diagnosis	Type of inflammatory cell	Generalized meningeal thickening	Meningeal cellular infiltration	Cortical nerve cell damage	Cortical gliosis	White matter gliosis	Glial nodules	Abscess formation	Intracellular inclusion bodies	Distribution of lesion	Extent of resection
15*	Meningitis/AHS	Small round cell	+	+	0	+	+	0	0	0	Widespread	Incomplete
48*	Meningitis/AHS	Mixed polymorph and small round cell	+	+	0	+	+	0	0	0	Widespread	Incomplete
193	Meningitis	Small round cell	+	+	0	+	+	0	0	0	Widespread	Incomplete
214	Meningitis	Mixed polymorph and small round cell	+	+	+	+	+	0	0	0	Widespread	Incomplete
249	Meningitis	Small round cell	+	+	0	+	+	0	0	0	Widespread	Incomplete

Neuropathology

Case No. Diagnosis	Type of inflammatory cell	Generalized meningeal thickening	Meningeal cellular infiltration	Cortical nerve cell damage	Cortical gliosis	White matter gliosis	Glial nodules	Abscess formation	Intracellular inclusion bodies	Distribution of lesion	Extent of resection
16* Abscess/AHS	Mixed polymorph and small round cell	0	0	+	+	+	+	+	+	(Fusiform & T3)	Total
62 Abscess	Mixed polymorph and small round cell	0	0	+	+	+	+	+	+	(T3)	Total
83 Abscess	Mixed polymorph and small round cell	0	0	+	+	+	+	+	+	(Fusiform, T3, T2)	Total
130 Encephalitis	Small round cell	0	+	+	+	+	+	0	0	Widespread	Incomplete
224 Abscess	Small round cell	+	+	+	+	+	+	+	+	(T3 & T2)	Total
247 Encephalitis	Small round cell	0	+	+	+	+	+	+	0	Widespread	Incomplete

*Double pathology
T2 = middle temporal gyrus   T3 = inferior temporal gyrus

GROUP 6. INDEFINITE

Twenty-five patients (17 male and 8 female)

Clinical results

Case No.	Age at operation	Sex	Birth injury	Febrile convulsions	Pre-op. fit frequency
	Age at first fit	Side of lobectomy	Head injury	Status epilepticus	Other
1	30y	F	0	0	+++
	13y	Right	0	0	0
14	33y	F	0	0	Not known
	17y	Left	+	0	0
23	14y	M	0	0	+++
	9y	Left	0	0	0
26	28y	M	0	0	Not known
	13y	Right	0	0	0
50	21y	M	+	0	++
	11y	Left	0	0	0
52	22y	M	0	0	++
	10y	Right	0	0	Schizophrenic
54	27y	M	0	0	+
	3y	Left	+	0	0
80	20y	F	0	0	+++
	13y	Left	0	0	0
86	31y	M	0	0	+
111	50y	M	0	0	+
	16y	Left	0	0	Aggressive
125	38y	M	0	0	+
	30y	Left	+	0	0
132	18y	F	0	+	+
	5y	Right	0	0	0
140	38y	M	0	0	+
	7y	Left	0	0	0
142	25y	M	0	0	+++
	7y	Left	+	0	0
150	42y	F	0	+	Not known
	4y	Right	0	0	0

Case No.	Age at operation	Sex	Birth injury	Febrile convulsions	Pre-op. fit frequency
	Age at first fit	Side of lobectomy	Head injury	Status epilepticus	Other comments
151	42y	F	0	0	+
	18y	Right	0	0	0
169	16y	M	0	0	+++
	2y	Right	+	0	Psychotic
178	28y	F	0	+	+
	1y	Right	0	+	0
192	37y	M	0	0	+++
	31y	Right	0	0	0
196	30y	M	+	0	+++
	12y	Left	0	0	0
199	47y	M	0	0	+++
	30y	Right	+	0	0
204	34y	F	0	0	+++
	21y	Right	0	0	0
221	34y	M	0	0	+
	30y	Left	0	0	0
233	37y	M	0	0	++
	10y	Right	+	0	0
242	39y	M	0	0	+++
	32y	Right	0	0	0

Number of cases: 25
Age range at operation: 14–50 years. Mean 31.24 years. S.D. 9.51
Age range at first fit: 1–35 years. Mean 14.72 years. S.D. 10.74

Post-operative results and neuropathology

Case No. Diagnosis	Length of follow-up	Fit frequency	Personality and social adjustment	Comments
1 Gliosis + ? neuronal abnormality	4y	Worse	Worse	Depressed and suicidal
14 Gliosis + ? scar	20y	Worse	Worse	Aggressive, demented, in-patient in mental hospital
23 ? recent cortical infarction	3y	Unaltered	Unaltered	Specimen incomplete
26 Gliosis	No f/u	—	—	—
50 ? old haemorrhage	6y	Worse	Worse	Died in status epilepticus Specimen incomplete
52 Gliosis	No f/u	—	—	—
54 ? glial anomaly in amygdala	14y	Fit-free	Normal life	Greatly improved Specimen incomplete

Post-operative results and neuropathology

Case No. Diagnosis	Length of follow-up	Fit frequency	Personality and social adjustment	Comments
80 Gliosis	16y	Unaltered	Unaltered	
86 Gliosis	1y	Unaltered	Unaltered	Specimen incomplete
111 Cuffed vessels in inferior horn	1y	Worse	Worse	Aggressive, in-patient in mental hospital
125 ? glial anomaly in amygdala	10y	Fit-free	Normal life	Greatly improved
132 Gliosis	7y	Unaltered	Unaltered	
140 ? glial anomaly in amygdala	21y	Improved	Improved	
142 Gliosis	15y	Fit-free	Normal life	Greatly improved
150 Gliosis	No f/u	—	—	Specimen incomplete

Patient / Histology	f/u			
151 Gliosis	14y	Unaltered	Worse	Schizophrenic Specimen incomplete
169 Gliosis	8y	Worse	Worse	Died in status epilepticus
178 Gliosis	16y	Improved	Unaltered	Specimen incomplete
192 Gliosis	15y	Fit-free	Unaltered	Specimen incomplete
196 Gliosis and localized meningeal thickening	18y	Fit-free	Unaltered	Specimen incomplete
199 Gliosis and ? neuronal loss	17y	Unaltered	Unaltered	Specimen incomplete
204 ? Glial abnormality	4y	Improved	Improved	
221 Gliosis	2y	Worse	Worse	Died – suicide
233 ? old haemorrhage	2y	Unaltered	Unaltered	
242 Gliosis	2y	Unaltered	Unaltered	

f/u = follow-up. Follow-up information available on 22 patients.
Average length of follow-up 10 years.
Effect of operation on fit pattern: Greatly improved (5), Improved (3), Unaltered (8), Worse (6)
Effect of operation on personality and social adjustment: Greatly improved (3), Improved (2), Unaltered (10), Worse (7)

GROUP 7.   NO APPARENT LESION

41 patients (26 male and 15 female)
Clinical results

Case No.	Age at operation	Sex	Birth injury	Febrile convulsions	Pre-op. fit frequency
	Age at first fit	Side of lobectomy	Head injury	Status epilepticus	Other
5	38y	M	0	0	+++
	27y	Left	0	0	Schizophrenic
9	25y	F	0	0	+++
	21y	Left	0	+	0
11	39y	F	0	0	Not known
	35y	Left	0	0	Narcoleptic
12	28y	F	0	0	++
	15y	Right	0	0	0
13	27y	F	0	0	+
	9y	Right	0	+	Schizophrenic
19	29y	M	+	0	Not known
	24y	Left	0	0	0
21	25y	F	0	0	+
	5y	Right	0	0	Aggressive
33	54y	M	0	0	+
	36y	Left	0	0	Psychotic
38	49y	M	0	0	+
	39y	Left	0	0	0
39	16y	F	0	0	+
	7y	Left	0	0	0
40	21y	M	0	0	++
	13y	Right	0	0	0
47	39y	F	0	0	+++
	27y	Left	+	0	Aggressive
51	51y	M	0	0	+
	47y	Right	0	0	0
64	12y	M	0	0	Not known
	3y	Left	0	0	0
70	42y	M	0	0	+++
	24y	Left	0	0	0

Case No.	Age at operation	Sex	Birth injury	Febrile convulsions	Pre-op. fit frequency
	Age at first fit	Side of lobectomy	Head injury	Status epilepticus	Other
77	13y	M	+	0	+++
	11y	Left	0	0	0
81	40y	M	0	0	+++
	28y	Right	0	+	0
92	12y	M	0	0	++
	11y	Left	0	0	Aggressive
97	42y	M	0	0	++
	27y	Left	0	0	0
108	20y	M	0	0	+++
	13y	Left	+	0	0
118	14y	F	+	0	+++
	Birth	Left	0	+	Mental defective
124	17y	M	0	0	++
	12y	Right	0	0	0
126	22y	M	0	0	+++
	1y	Right	+	0	0
127	27y	M	0	0	+++
	5y	Right	0	0	0
134	9y	M	0	0	+++
	7y	Left	0	0	0
138	42y	M	0	0	+
	38y	Left	0	0	Aggressive/ schizophrenic
146	28y	M	0	0	+++
	12y	Left	0	0	0
158	20y	F	0	0	++
	11y	Right	0	+	0
167	24y	M	0	0	++
	2y	Right	0	0	0
177	17y	F	0	0	+
	7y	Right	+	0	0

Case No.	Age at operation	Sex	Birth injury	Febrile convulsions	Pre-op. fit frequency
	Age at first fit	Side of lobectomy	Head injury	Status epilepticus	Other
179*	25y & 27y	M	+	0	+++
	19y	Right & Left	0	0	0
180	32y	M	0	0	+++
	17y	Left	0	0	0
185	17y	M	0	0	++
	6y	Left	0	0	Aggressive
200	22y	F	0	0	++
	16y	Right	0	0	0
210	38y	M	0	0	++
	7y	Right	0	0	Aggressive
212	41y	M	0	0	+
	20y	Right	+	0	0
219	21y	F	0	+	+++
	2y	Left	0	0	0
222	27y	M	0	0	++
	14y	Left	0	0	0
225	38y	F	0	0	++
	8y	Left	0	0	Depressed
231	27y	F	0	0	Not known
	20y	Left	0	0	0
248	45y	F	0	0	++
	7y	Left	0	0	Schizophrenic

*Patient No. 179 underwent bilateral temporal lobectomy and died one year after operation.
Age range at operation: 9–54 years. Mean 28.56 years. S.D. 11.78
Age range at first fit: Birth–47 years. Mean 15.37 years. S.D. 11.68

Post-operative results

Case No.	Length of follow-up	Fit frequency	Personality and social adjustment	Comments
5	3y	Fit-free	Unaltered	Still schizophrenic Impotent
9	12y	Improved	Unaltered	Depressed
11	10y	Improved	Unaltered	Still narcoleptic
12	9y	Worse	Worse	Aggressive
13	3y	Improved	Unaltered	Still schizophrenic, also depressed
19	1y	Fit-free	Worse	Suicidal
21	No f/u			
33	11y	Unaltered	Unaltered	Depressed, aggressive and psychotic
38	17y	Improved	Improved	
39	1y	Unaltered	Unaltered	
40	9y	Fit-free	Normal life	Greatly improved
47	2y	Improved	Normal life	
51	14y	Fit-free	Unaltered	Post-op. hemiplegia, recurrent depression
64	No f/u			
70	1y	Fit-free	Improved	
77	10y	Worse	Worse	Intractable personality disorder
81	18y	Fit-free	Normal life	Greatly improved
92	10y	Worse	Worse	Aggressive and depressed
97	7y	Worse	Worse	Aggressive
108	8y	Worse	Unaltered	
118	2y	Worse	Worse	Died – anaemia, cerebral thrombosis
124	No f/u	–	–	–
126	7y	Worse	Worse	Subsequent leucotomy. Frequently depressed and suicidal

Case No.	Length of follow-up	Fit frequency	Personality and social adjustment	Comments
127	12y	Worse	Worse	Subsequent leucotomy. Frequently depressed and suicidal
134	3y	Unaltered	Unaltered	
138	1y	Worse	Worse	Died – suicide
146	4y	Worse	Worse	Depressed
158	7y	Worse	Worse	Frontal leucotomy after 7 yrs – much improved
167	1y	Unaltered	Unaltered	
177	4y	Worse	Worse	Aggressive, schizophrenic
179	2y	Worse	Worse	Died in status
	1y	Worse	Worse	epilepticus
180	16y	Improved	Worse	
185	3y	Worse	Worse	Died in status epilepticus
200	12y	Fit-free	Normal life	Greatly improved
210	1y	Unaltered	Unaltered	
212	4 mths	Unaltered	Unaltered	Died in a fit
219	18y	Unaltered	Unaltered	
222	16y	Fit-free	Normal life	Greatly improved
225	15y	Fit-free	Improved	
231	11y	Fit-free	Worse	Ataxic
248	20y	Fit-free	Worse	Still schizophrenic and alcoholic

f/u = follow up.
Follow-up information available on 38 patients.
Effect of operation on fit Pattern:
   Greatly improved (8), Improved (9), Unaltered (7), Worse (14)
Effect of operation on personality and social adjustment:
   Greatly improved (4). Improved (4), Unaltered (13), Worse (17)

Neuropathology
By definition, all the temporal lobes in this group appeared completely normal.

GROUP 8. DOUBLE PATHOLOGY

18 patients (10 male and 8 female)

Clinical results

The clinical and neuropathological details of each case have been itemized in the relevant diagnostic groups but a summary of these is given below:
Age range at operation: 9–36 yrs.   Mean 22.33 yrs. S.D. 6.83
Age range at first fit: 8 mths–35 yrs. Mean 9.53 yrs. S.D. 8.75

Post-operative results

Follow-up on 17 patients. Average length of follow-up: 9 years.
Effect of operation on fit pattern:
    Greatly improved (8), Improved (6), Unaltered (1), Worse (2)
Effect of operation on personality and social adjustment:
    Greatly improved (5), Improved (2), Unaltered (5), Worse (5)
The complete abnormality was considered to have been removed in 16 of the 18 cases. The remaining two specimens (Case Nos. 15 and 48) showed the presence of a widespread inflammatory process which was thought unlikely to be confined to the temporal lobe.

Neuropathology

Case No.	Neuropathological diagnosis
4	AHS+Cortical scar
10	AHS+Neuronoglial lesion
15	AHS+Inflammatory lesion
16	AHS+Inflammatory lesion
28	AHS+Vascular lesion
48	AHS+Inflammatory lesion
55	AHS+Cortical scar
57	AHS+Developmental cyst
60	AHS+Neuronoglial lesion
98	Developmental cyst+Neuronoglial lesion
131	AHS+Oligodendroglial lesion
137	Developmental cyst + Mixed glial lesion
144	AHS+Neuronoglial lesion
147	AHS+Astrocytic glial lesion
164	Developmental cyst+Mixed glial lesion
207	AHS+Mixed glial lesion
227	AHS+Cortical scar
240	AHS+Mixed glial lesion

Distribution of the lesion
The most frequently damaged areas were the 'mesial temporal' structures where the hippocampus was involved in 15 cases. The amygdaloid nucleus (14 cases). the uncus (10 cases) and the parahippocampal gyrus (8 cases) were also commonly involved.

Index